MIDWEST
MEDICINAL
PLANTS

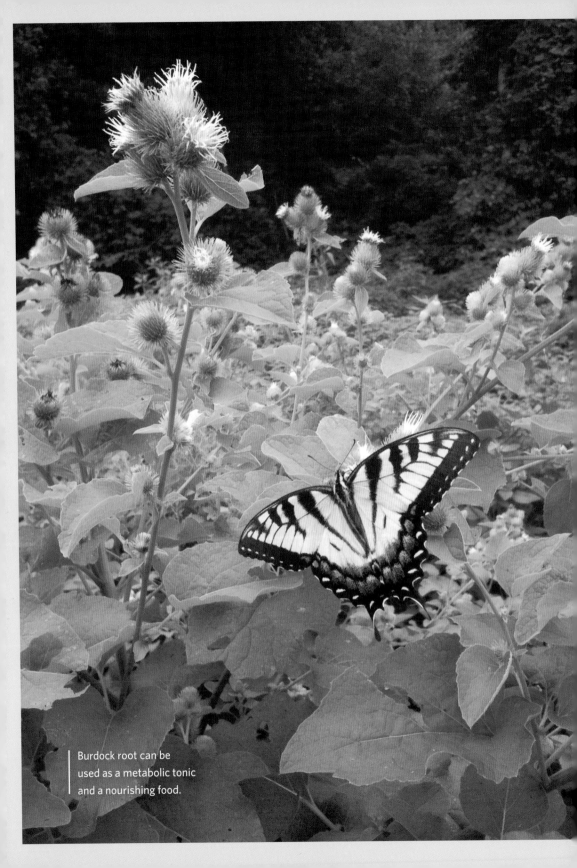

Burdock root can be used as a metabolic tonic and a nourishing food.

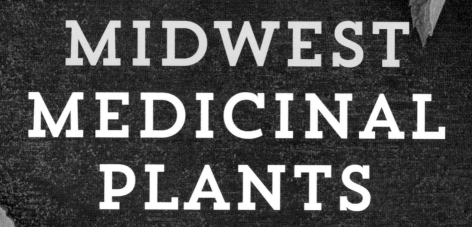

MIDWEST
MEDICINAL
PLANTS

IDENTIFY, HARVEST, AND USE
⚜ 109 WILD HERBS ⚜
FOR HEALTH AND WELLNESS

LISA M. ROSE

The information in this book is true and complete to the best of
our knowledge. All recommendations are made without guarantee
on the part of the author or Timber Press. The author and publisher
disclaim any liability in connection with the use of this information.
In particular, ingesting wild plants and fungi is inherently risky.
Plants can be easily mistaken and individuals vary in their
physiological reactions to plants that are touched or consumed.
Please do not attempt self-treatment of a medical problem without
consulting a qualified health practitioner.

Published in 2017 by Timber Press, Inc.
The Haseltine Building
133 S.W. Second Avenue, Suite 450
Portland, Oregon 97204-3527
timberpress.com

Printed in China
Sixth printing 2021
Text and cover design by Adrianna Sutton

Library of Congress Cataloging-in-Publication Data
Names: Rose, Lisa M. (Herbalist) author.
Title: Midwest medicinal plants : identify, harvest, and use 109 wild herbs for
    health and wellness / Lisa M. Rose.
Description: Portland, Oregon: Timber Press, 2017. | Includes bibliographical
    references and index.
Identifiers: LCCN 2016045510 (print) | LCCN 2016049723 (ebook) | ISBN
    9781604696554 (pbk.) | ISBN 9781604698138 (e-book)
Subjects: LCSH: Medicinal plants—Middle West. | Herbs—Therapeutic use—
    Middle West. | Materia medica, Vegetable—Middle West.
Classification: LCC RS180.L3 R67 2017 (print) | LCC RS180.L3 (ebook) | DDC
    615.3/21—dc23 LC record available at https://lccn.loc.gov/2016045510

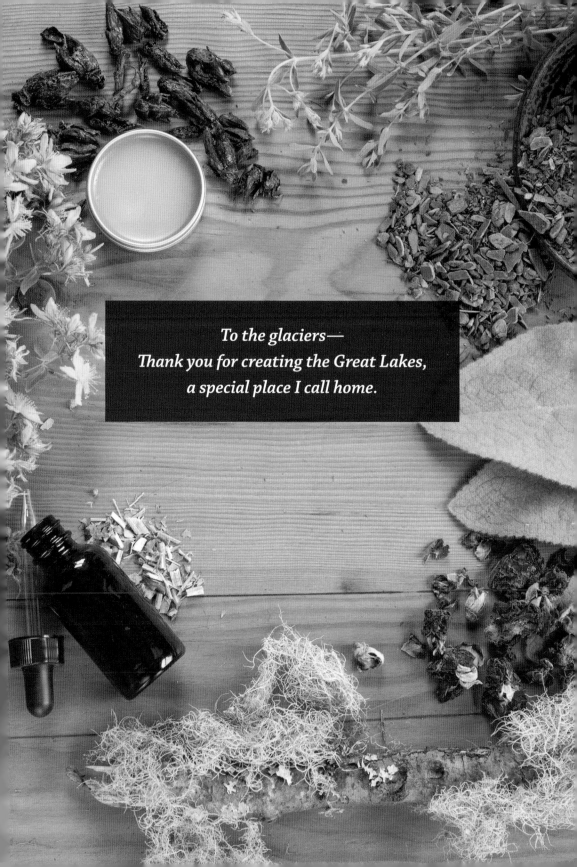

To the glaciers—
Thank you for creating the Great Lakes,
a special place I call home.

CONTENTS

PREFACE
GROWING AN HERBALIST

If the earth needs an herbalist, it will grow one.
— jim mcdonald, Great Lakes herbalist, 2010

first turned to the plants for guidance at the age of 30. Although I'd always been a plant person, I'd been working against nature's cycles and against my own. I was worn out, tired from the cultural stress that I was carrying from running an NGO, being a mom to two small kids, and being a good wife.

A gardener, I was even too tired to plant seeds in the springtime or clear away the winter's debris. "Maybe you shouldn't clear away the debris or plant anything this year," a wise farmer friend told me. "Maybe you should just listen to the plants and see what they have to say."

This was the beginning of my practice as an herbalist. I sat down and began to listen to the plants. I let my garden go fallow and watched the land take over in the way that it knows how to do.

My interests in gardening slowly transformed into working nearly entirely with wild plants. I noticed the weeds growing between the cultivated plants and between

the cracks in the sidewalk. I wondered about their resilience and their potential healing powers. I learned their names and how they tasted, smelled, and felt in my fingers.

Burdock called to me from the ditches of my friend's farm. Burdock would become the first plant I'd work with as an herbal medicine. And my apothecary grew, as did a need for my teachings in my community.

I was called to be a teacher in 2010 by my own teacher, Jim McDonald. "Lisa Rose, if it looks like a duck and quacks like a duck, it's a duck," said Jim. "You work with wild plants. You make plant medicines. You share them with others. You, in fact, are an herbalist."

From that point forward, I opened my

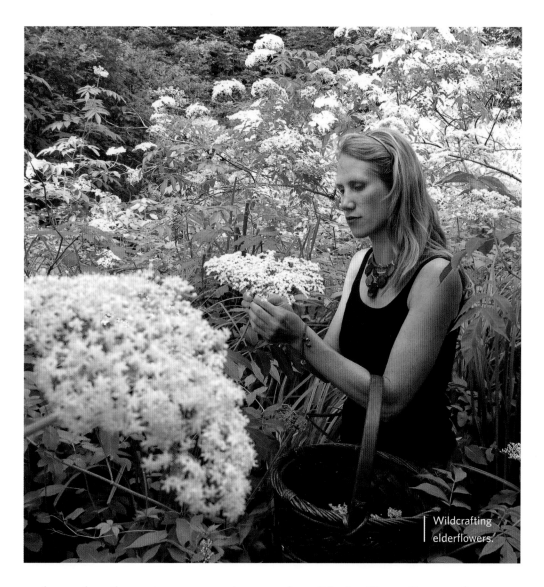

Wildcrafting elderflowers.

gardens and apothecary to my community. Jim and others sent clients my way for my practice. I was scared that I didn't know enough. But instead of being stuck in that rut, I stepped forward to teach what I knew. Since that time, I've never really looked back. And with an insatiable curiosity, I've never stopped being a student of the plants.

You will find that this book is filled with nuggets of learning that I've acquired across a delicious and healing journey with the plants. It's what I know. Ten years from now, I hope to know more, layered upon this foundation.

In your herbal journey, I encourage you to start with what you know. Go outside and listen to the plants. Touch, taste, smell, and repeat. Get to know the plants on an intimate level. And share this love with everyone you know.

You are an herbalist, and the earth needs you.

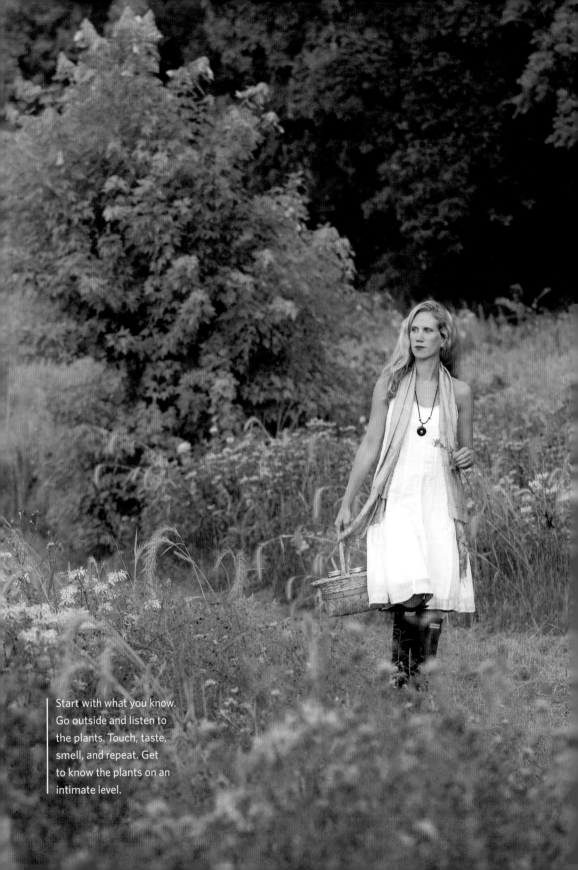

Start with what you know. Go outside and listen to the plants. Touch, taste, smell, and repeat. Get to know the plants on an intimate level.

WILDCRAFTING BASICS

Imagine this at the end of your harvest season: your own herbal apothecary, filled with local plants and herbs that you can turn to as you feel a cold coming on or notice a stomach upset after an indulgent meal. There is nothing more gratifying than to know that you can keep yourself and your family healthy throughout the year with the plant-based medicines you've created from the wild plants you've gathered, or wildcrafted, from the fields, hedgerows, and woodlands around you.

For many, an herbal apothecary evokes images of shelves full of bottles and jars filled with mysterious herbs and herbal formulas from exotic plants. But to create an herbal apothecary that your family can turn to for basic ills and chills, you don't need to include exotic or mysterious plants. In fact, as you realize that you can incorporate local plants and herbs into your natural wellness routines, you can begin to create a personal apothecary using plants that grow just outside your front stoop.

All you need to do is pay attention to the plants growing around you. This will help you connect to the land and nature itself—even as you're engulfed by our manic, developed world. Eating wild foods and using plant medicines created from the fruits of the earth will bind you to a place—its rivers, animals, smells, sights, and sounds. Ingesting these fruits makes a place literally a part of you, so that the land and its story become your story—a story of the earth, people, politics, and infrastructure all bound together by an invisible red thread. It is healing, this wild medicine.

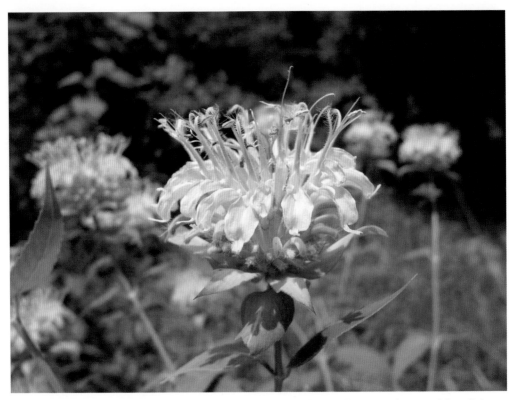

Monarda fistulosa, wild bergamot, is often incorporated into landscape designs and is a useful medicine.

As herbalists, we are land stewards. Working with wild plants requires that we understand not just their botany, but their abundance and impact in our bioregion. We should know whether a plant is endangered (and should not be wildcrafted) or invasive (which can be the best to wildcraft from a sustainability standpoint). We should know how to wildcraft a plant in the most careful way so that it can continue to reproduce for future harvests and enjoyment.

Know and pay attention to the bounty (or lack thereof) that's around you. This information should guide you first and foremost in your wildcrafting. Get to know the various habitats that surround you. Plant populations vary in each habitat, from hardwood deciduous forests, to wetlands, to urban lots. Over time, you will know intimately the microclimates and plant life in your area, including which plants might be threatened or limited in amount.

HOW TO USE THIS BOOK ON YOUR JOURNEY

Use this book to hone your skills as both a wildcrafter and medicine-maker. Both new and experienced herbalists will find this guide to be a useful addition to their medicine-making toolkits. Those who are simply interested in greening up their kitchens and medicine kits will also find plenty of information about exploring a hyperlocal source for plant-based remedies for everyday wellness needs.

Within each plant profile in the book, I discuss how to harvest the plants safely to avoid negatively impacting the plant

Know Thy Plants: Safe and Respectful Harvesting

It is wise, for a multitude of reasons, to identify the plants correctly before you do any handling, wildcrafting, or tasting. Do not harvest a plant unless you are sure you can identify it correctly. Harvesting a plant without knowing what you have is disrespectful of both the plant and you: you can get seriously ill from wildcrafting and ingesting the wrong plant. Safety first: poisoning is both possible and a serious health risk. Don't try to cheat your way through plant identification. If you think a plant *might* be safe, do not harvest or eat it until you *know* it is safe. It's easy, and a bad idea, to skip over the details and make a plant fit a description even if some details don't match perfectly.

population. Remember to do no harm, and leave the places in which you harvest better than when you found them.

Your Herbal Harvest

This book provides descriptions of 109 medicinal plants that grow and can be harvested in the Midwest. It guides you through the seasons to help you identify plants to use for medicine-making, including when and how to wildcraft and prepare them.

In each plant profile, you will learn how to identify the plant; where, when, and how to wildcraft it; how it can be used as medicine; and why its medicinal action is helpful for optimal health. Each profile also includes suggestions regarding how to prepare and use the plant and its part as herbal medicine.

Wild and weedy plants are resilient and tolerate tough growing conditions. Invasive weeds make up most of the herbs in my herbal apothecary, and I include many of my favorites in this book. In addition to the weeds, many medicinal plants, such as echinacea and wild bergamot, can be incorporated beautifully into any landscape design.

I encourage you to give up your lawn and allow that space to "rewild" itself into lush ecosystems filled with wild plants that you can use in your apothecary. Plant profiles make special mention of whether a plant is suited to an edible landscape or permaculture landscape plan. This will help you be mindful of the sustainability of plant populations so the land can continue to nourish us for years to come.

Safety is always at the fore when preparing and consuming wild plants. The plants included in this guide for use as medicinal remedies are the plants I use in my family's apothecary and with my community in my herbal practice. Any need for caution or other concerns in harvesting or using a plant are mentioned at the end of each profile. And remember that you must always be certain in your identification.

In addition, with introducing any new plant-based food to your body, you should do so with proper care to eliminate the potential for adverse reactions. Not all plants are a match for all people. It is your responsibility to learn more about individual plants and how they work with your needs and your body.

Tasting and smelling your freshly harvested herbs will set you on your way to understanding how plants can be used in times of illness and as part of your regular diet. Notice and compare how dry herbs and fresh plants taste fresh and in tea. You will learn ways to prepare the herbs to suit your tastes and medicinal needs. As you continue along your herbal harvest journey, experiment with single herbs or try blending them.

To hone your herbalism skills, seek out a multitude of resources. Near the end of the book are recommendations on good sources of information, herbal remedies, and plants.

What Regions Are Included

Those living across the Midwestern states, including Illinois, Indiana, Iowa, Kansas, Michigan, Minnesota, Missouri, Nebraska, North Dakota, Ohio, South Dakota, and Wisconsin, will find this book helpful. Canadians in the immediate region of Ontario will also find relevant information here.

The included plants grow across most of the Midwest's ecologically diverse bioregions, from the prairies, to the woodlands, to the dunes habitats on the shores of the Great Lakes. With a focus on safety, prudence, and biodiversity, this book will help you identify areas that are safe and suitable for wildcrafting.

INTO THE WILD

As an herbalist, I am frequently asked, "What's growing outside now that I can wildcraft? How do I know which plants can be used medicinally?"

The best way to determine which plants to wildcraft is to pay attention to the plants that grow around you. You can rely on these wild plants for medicine. Step right outside your door to start learning. With a field guide, sketchbook, and perhaps a camera in hand, you can document the plants that you see.

Create your own map of your area, and check Google Maps, taking note of the significant natural structures in the landscape, such as lakes, streams, and forests, and man-made constructs, such as highways, factories, buildings, and the like. Use this map as a tool, taking it along on regular walks. Bring a friend, your kids, or a neighbor, and talk about what you notice.

As you notice plants, add them to your map. Take photos of the plants to remember their physical characteristics, or use colored pencils and paper to sketch discoveries along your route. Take plant cuttings if you need to. Make note of the weather, time of day, and time of year. You don't need to get caught up in learning plant names at first. Collect your photos, drawings, and cuttings and start your identification process using them for reference.

Do all of this before you wildcraft any plants.

Get Permission First

If you want to wildcraft any plants in areas beyond your own property, remember that laws protect privately owned property and public areas such as parks from unauthorized wildcrafting and trespassing. Poaching, the illegal taking of wild plants or animals, is a serious problem, so get the appropriate permissions to enter and wildcraft in an area before you go there. On private property, ask the owner to go along with you—you might even make a new friend!

People in many cultures and native traditions who work with wild plants also reverently ask the plant for permission to harvest it. If you do this with a sense of respect and gratitude, there is always an answer from the plant. We can choose to ask and listen.

Gear for the Field

As a wildcrafter, you need the appropriate tools to help you comfortably and successfully gather wild plants and get them back to the kitchen for cleaning and preservation. Your toolkit will vary depending on the plants you want to harvest. Some of the plant profiles in this book note specific tools you may need for the harvest, but in general,

BASIC LEAF ARRANGEMENTS AND SHAPES

Botanical nomenclature can be somewhat intimidating. The language used in this book is intended to be functional and accessible to avoid too much technical botanical terminology.

After you have spent time observing plants, you will be able to identify key botanical features such as leaves, reproductive parts, and flowers more easily. For starters, knowing and using the appropriate botanical language to identify a few leaf arrangements and shapes can help in your identification. Seek out additional botanical resources at the end of the book to expand your knowledge.

ALTERNATE

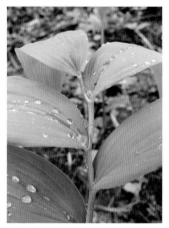

The leaves of Solomon's seal grow in an alternate pattern along the stem.

COMPOUND WITH LEAFLETS

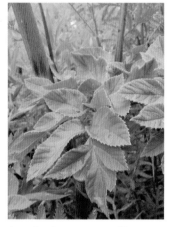

Angelica has compound leaves, each comprising several leaflets.

BASAL ROSETTE

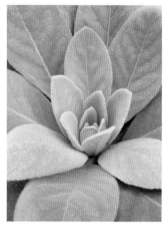

The leaves of the mullein form a basal rosette.

TOOTHED, LANCE-SHAPED

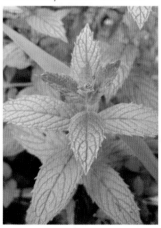

Spearmint leaves are toothed and lance-shaped.

OPPOSITE

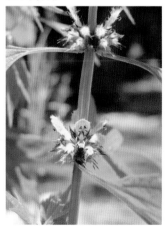

Motherwort leaves are arranged oppositely along the square stem.

WHORLED

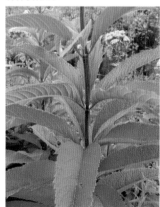

Joe Pye weed leaves grow in a circular whorled pattern up the stem.

any wildcrafting kit should contain several items.

Hand tools Digging forks, small hand trowel, loppers, hori, kitchen shears, pruners, handsaw, and leather gloves

Specialty tools Nut gatherer (a rolling tool used to pick up nuts), nutcracker, and tweezers

Containers Berry baskets, shallow trays, buckets, burlap sacks, cotton market bags of various sizes, and paper lunch sacks for smaller harvests

Botanical identification materials Plant identification books, camera, sketch pad, hand loupe, ruler, scissors, and small plastic or paper bags for gathering samples of plants to identify at your desk

Clothing Techware outdoor wear or other lightweight clothing, shoes, socks, long pants to tuck into socks

Bug spray Herbal bug spray you create yourself

CONTAMINATION: NOT ALL SOILS AND PLANTS ARE EQUAL

As a city-dweller, I take soil contamination seriously. The soils in urban areas, particularly, can contain excess lead or other pollutants that can be absorbed by plant roots. Using contaminated water for irrigation can also affect concentrations of contaminants in the plants.

Home gardeners can have their garden soils tested before planting, but most herbalists wildcrafting plants won't be soil testing in areas where they are collecting and harvesting. To help ensure that you avoid wildcrafting in contaminated areas, know the history of the land where you want to wildcraft and what possible contaminants may be present. Ask the landowner and neighbors, and/or study public records, to determine whether contamination has been identified

in the soils or whether potential contaminating factors, such as gas stations or railway yards, have existed there or nearby. If you are uncertain of the area's use history, consider finding a different wildcrafting location.

Before wildcrafting in an area, carefully consider a variety of factors that could affect the quality and consumability of the plants.

Suburban pollution Excess residual herbicides and pesticides may be present in lawns, golf courses, roadsides, and corporate landscapes. Lead-based paint chips from older home and building exteriors can also accumulate in and contaminate the soil.

Urban pollution Heavy metals such as lead, arsenic, and other industrial

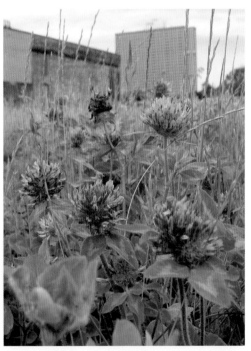

Red clover grows in an abandoned industrial lot in Detroit. Because of the likelihood of heavy metal contaminants (potentially lead) in the soil, I would avoid collecting these plants in urban lots, where they can absorb minerals and heavy metals from contaminated soil.

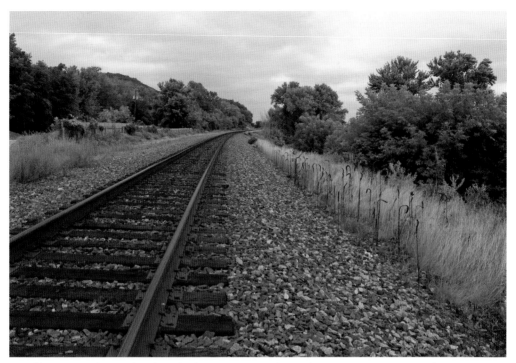

Avoid harvesting along railroad tracks, because surrounding soils may contain arsenic and creosote, which can be absorbed by plants.

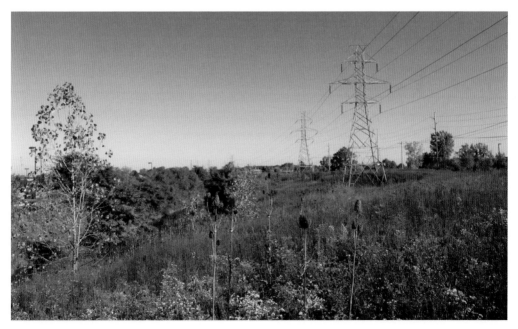

Herbicides are often used on easements to maintain clear access to power lines and other municipal services.

pollutants may be present in areas that were once heavily industrialized, such as current brownfields (zones of heavily polluted areas, as designated by the Environmental Protection Agency or Canadian Department of the Environment); old refuse and landfill sites; railroad tracks (arsenic) and roundhouse areas; highways; and old gas station sites.

Agricultural pollution Rural soils can contain as many contaminants as urban soils. Farms can be sources of excess nitrates, fertilizers, and manure runoff. The presence of manure adds a possible source of watershed contamination such as *E. coli* and *Salmonella*. This is particularly important when you are considering plants that grow in wetlands or in a riverbed that is downstream from a farm or feedlot.

Corporate pollution Pharmaceutical companies, manufacturing complexes, the furniture industry, and paint companies are all potential environmental polluters, especially with regard to heavy metals.

Municipal pollution At water treatment facilities, sewage overflow can contribute to *E. coli* and *Salmonella* loads in surrounding soils and waterways. Power facilities may dump residual by-products (including gray water) into nearby waterways.

Public easement pollution Herbicides are often used on easements to kill plants and maintain clear access to power lines and other municipal services. The public is not usually notified when these easements are treated; it may be easy to spot herbicidal treatment areas, however, because they are often brown and appear to have been burned.

Roadway pollution In winter, icy roads are often treated with a salt or bromide solution, and increasingly popular is the use of fracking wastewater as a deicer. These chemicals may be absorbed by surrounding

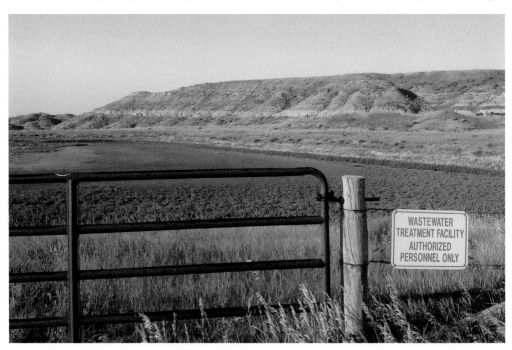

Know which way the water flows. Gray irrigation water from wastewater treatment plants can be contaminated with waterborne pathogens such as *E. coli* and *Salmonella*.

Heavy Metal Contamination of Plants

Any plant that we eat for its mineral content (such as dock, lamb's quarters, and nettle) can take up and synthesize heavy metals, such as lead, from the soil. Because dock roots take up and store iron, for example, the plant may be predisposed to absorb other minerals that may be unhealthy in quantity to the human body, such as lead or arsenic. If curly or yellow dock grows in an area where commercial manufacturing has occurred, it can contain contaminants drawn from the soil and should be avoided.

Not all plants and plant parts absorb contaminants in the same way. Seeds of dock may have a different concentration of lead than roots, for example, because the roots are in direct contact with the soil and any contaminants contained within it. There is no rule of thumb that indicates whether a plant is safe or unsafe, but knowing how a plant can be affected by soil contaminants helps you know what is possible for the plant and what you should be looking for as you wildcraft.

If there is ever any question or doubt as to potential contamination, move along and do not gather the plant.

plant material, which appears burned and dead during the growing season.

Irrigated land pollution Gray water used in irrigation can be contaminated with waterborne bacteria. Washing plants in water cannot eliminate all pathogens, such as *E. coli* and *Salmonella*.

THE HERBALIST'S APOTHECARY

You may find that you like wildcrafting and working with plants so much that you will want to delve into making herbal teas, salves, infused oils, and tinctures. You will discover that it is truly satisfying to begin to rely on the natural world for wellness and to connect to a tradition of herbal healing and reliance on plants that is as old as human history.

The Well-Stocked Pantry

When you return home with your harvest in hand, you'll need a well-stocked pantry to process your harvest into plant medicines. Being prepared will ensure that your hard efforts in the field won't spoil on the counter waiting to be processed and preserved. Have the right pantry staples on hand to help keep your bounty fresh. Raw honey, for example, is a prime staple in my own pantry for helping preserve my wild harvests.

It's also in every herbalist's interest to keep costs low in acquiring and replenishing medicine-making tools. You can procure second-hand equipment such as funnels, ladles, measuring cups, and jars (new lids are required with each new batch of preserves). Resale shops, garage and estate sales, and even grandmas' kitchens are great sources of gadgets to help round out your preservation kit.

A well-stocked preservation pantry should include a number of staples:

- apothecary bottles, various sizes
- canners, pans, teakettle
- canning jars with new sealing lids
- dehydrator
- drying screens
- funnels
- grinder, mortar and pestle
- homebrew supplies such as carboys

(large jugs), buckets, siphons, thermo-meter, yeasts
- liquors such as grape liquors, mead, mescal, tequila, vodka, wine
- olive oil
- paper bags
- raw honey
- salts such as pickling salt, rock salt, sea salt
- sugar
- tongs, ladles, spoons
- twine
- vinegars

Cleaning and Storing Plant Material

Before they are used or dried, all plant parts should be thoroughly and carefully cleaned to remove debris, dust, soil, and insects. To dry plant material after cleaning, place individual flowers, leaves, stems, or root pieces on screens in a dry location, or use a dehydrator. Bundle larger plant stalks and hang them to dry in a well-ventilated, dry location.

Harvest the plants after the morning dew has evaporated to reduce the amount of water on the materials, and make sure that the plant material is fully dry before you store it in clean glass jars. Any moisture in the material will mold in the jar and cannot be used.

In addition, always label and date the jars in which you store your herbal harvests. Dried aromatic plant materials can usually be kept for use for a year or, sometimes, two years. To test the vitality of stored plant materials, crumble them between your fingers. If they are still aromatic, they are still usable and viable.

Plants and herbs can sometimes be stored in the refrigerator or freezer as well. This option, when appropriate for particular plants or plant parts, is indicated in specific plant profiles.

Preserving Food Safely

Before any food preservation begins, you'll need a basic working knowledge of food safety, handling, and processing. The US Department of Agriculture offers a free online resource with a complete index on canning and processing at the National Center for Home Food Preservation (nchfp.uga.edu). You will find lots of good information about setting up your kitchen for proper food handling and safely processing food and herbs.

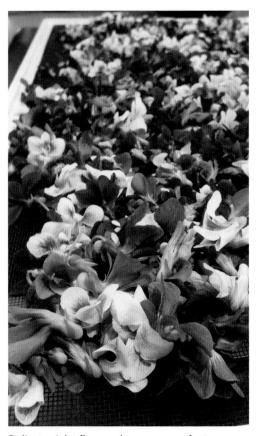

Delicate violet flowers dry on screens for tea. Drying screens are useful for drying flowers, leaves, and stalks for teas.

MAKING PLANT MEDICINES

You can use fresh or dry plant material to create infusions, decoctions, teas, tinctures, oils, salves, and other medicines. But medicinal plants can be used many other ways. Two of the easiest herbal preparations to create are infusions and decoctions. Both can be used in teas or for external washes, or they can be poured into the bath. Boil them on the stove for a steam inhalation, or crush them and use them topically on the skin. There are so many ways to use plants! Consider the plants as your paints and the kitchen as your studio.

Infusions and Decoctions

For each herbal tea preparation in the book, I include whether an infusion or a decoction is best. The plant parts listed at the beginning

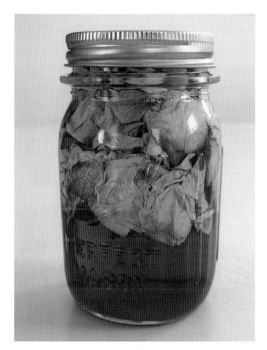

Plant petals, leaves, and other parts can be extracted in vinegars to make mineral-dense plant extracts. Here, rose petals are extracted in vinegar for a soothing skin spray.

of each plant profile should be used in the preparations unless others are specified.

An infusion involves steeping, or infusing, herbs in hot (hot infusion) or cold (cold infusion) water for a period of time. The preference for hot or cold water is herb-dependent and also dependent on what medicinal action is preferred. Infusions and decoctions can be consumed as tea, used topically as a wash, or used in a compress by soaking fabric or cotton balls in the infusion, squeezing out the excess moisture, and applying the material directly to the affected area.

COLD INFUSION

To make a cold infusion, use about 1 ounce of herbs and 32 ounces of water. Place the herbs in a tea ball or muslin bag in a glass or ceramic container. After one or two days, squeeze the bag of herbs into the water and add more water if necessary, depending on your taste preference.

You can also make a cold infusion similar to how to you would make sun tea. Place the water and herbs outside in the sun and allow them to infuse for a day or two, until the tea reaches the strength you prefer.

HOT INFUSION

Many herbs are easily infused in hot water for a few minutes in a tea ball in a cup or in a teapot or French press, and then poured into a cup to be enjoyed as a tea or wash. Hot water temperatures can extract more nutrients and other properties from the plant tissues. The amount of herbs and water depends on your preference with regard to the strength of the infusion.

DECOCTIONS

A decoction is a longer steep of the herbs in water, usually while over heat, and generally for 20 minutes or more. A decoction is best used to extract minerals from plant material. A decoction is simple to prepare: add the water and plant materials and simmer for 20–30 minutes.

Tinctures

Tinctures are liquid plant essences usually extracted in a base of alcohol. Start with either fresh or dry plant material along with a liquid solvent (called menstruum in herbal medicine)—often vodka or brandy. A high-proof grain alcohol, mead, wine, or vinegar can also be used, depending on the desired final product.

In selecting your menstruum, remember that high-proof alcohol will best extract plant resins, and vinegars will best extract plant minerals. In most cases for the home herbalist, using an affordable 50-percent alcohol (100-proof) vodka is perfectly acceptable to make common herbal tinctures.

To make a tincture, start by breaking down the plant material you want to tincture—for example, chop roots, cut up leafy plants, grind aromatic seeds, or crush berries. Then pack the plant material into a canning jar to 50 percent of its volume if the material is fresh or 25 percent if the material is dry.

Completely submerge the material and top off the jar with your chosen menstruum. To prevent unwanted spoilage, stir the plant material and menstruum to ensure that all the air bubbles escape. Cover, shake, and store the container in a dark place for a few weeks to allow full extraction of the plant's constituents.

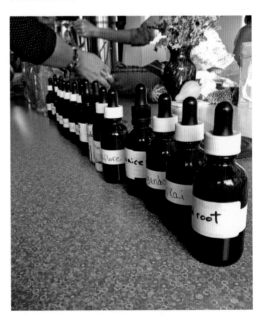

Tinctures are a staple of an herbalist's apothecary and a portable way to preserve plants as medicines.

Strain the finished extract into bottles. Alcohol-based plant extracts have a shelf life of three or more years if they are stored in a cool, dark place.

Infused Honey

Honey is a culinary staple that should be used frequently in place of refined, processed sugars (its glycemic index is about half that of white sugar). Local, raw honey is a truly pure medicine made by honey bees from plants and flowers that grow around us.

One of my favorite preparations of honey in both my kitchen and apothecary is to infuse it with local herbs. Using straight honey to soothe a cough or cold is easy and beneficial, but there is nothing more divine that spooning out raw honey that has been infused with beautiful herbs and flowers for several weeks. The flowers and plants impart not only their heavenly aromas, but their medicinal properties as well.

Infusing honey is a simple process. Gather leaves and flowers and add them to a jar. Then cover the herbs with honey and let the mixture infuse for several weeks in a cool, dark place, occasionally turning the jar upside down to blend the mixture. When you are ready to use the infused honey, strain out the herbs or let them remain—it's up to you.

Herbs that work well in infused honey include spotted bee balm, blue vervain, chamomile, elderflower, the invasive (and loved by me) honeysuckle, jasmine, lavender, lovage, mint, rose, and wild bergamot—but these are just a few of the possibilities. Onion and garlic are also great choices that make an excellent base for cough and cold syrups. I prefer to use fresh plant materials in season, but packaged organic herbs from

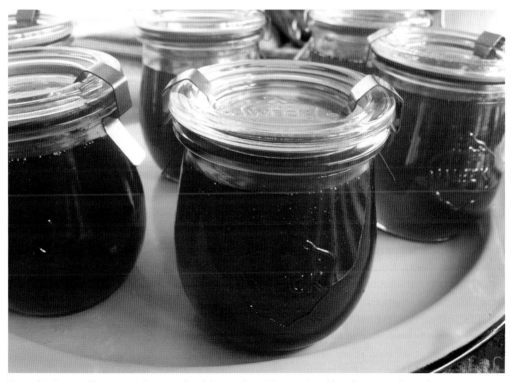

Every kitchen and home apothecary should never be without a jar of locally sourced, raw honey.

The Local Honey Pot

Sourcing local honey, like sourcing local food, is a good way to connect producers to consumers in your area and helps support beekeepers (and honey bees) in your community. It is easier than ever to find raw honey from a local beekeeper: visit a farmers' market or go online to LocalHarvest.org to find a supplier nearby. Honey that comes from local bees is created with the help of plants immediate to your growing area, which can help support your immune system, especially with regard to plant allergies.

Raw honey that hasn't been heat pasteurized (most commercially sold honey is pasteurized) also contains beneficial enzymes and is usually unfiltered. This means it can have a bigger (and better, in my opinion) aroma and flavor profile representative of the local flora. Local raw honey reflects the natural *terroir* (the particular qualities of the growing area) and has higher medicinal impact.

Because of the global food trade and economy, much of the commercial honey available at the supermarket comes from Brazil, China, and other faraway places. Large honey producers often blend batches from various regions. And, worse yet, some commercial honey is actually mixed with high fructose corn syrup, so it's not even real honey!

the market or dried plant material can also be used.

Because honey has antimicrobial and preservative qualities, the plant material in the infusion will not rot during the infusing process. There is a chance, however, that the herbs and honey will begin to ferment—which will be apparent if the mixture produces carbon dioxide and causes the lid to bulge—or worse, explode off the jar. In this case, you are well on your way to making mead. Contact a local brew shop for support on how to create this fine fermented concoction.

Add infused honey to herbal teas or eat it regularly to help support the body's immune responses to illness. Note, however, that eating honey is not a replacement for foundational immune strengthening: remember that diet, exercise, stress reduction, and sleep are core elements to staying healthy.

Other uses for infused honey include herbal truffles and slippery elm pastilles (lozenges). Create these wonderful honey-based preparations in large batches and then refrigerate them to have on hand to soothe a sore throat or stomachache. Using infused honey can make these creations especially delicious.

Infused honey can also serve as a base for herbal elixirs. I use it to make a delicious elderberry elixir. It offers not only the medicinal power of the plants and honey, but a nice flavor profile to this important apothecary staple.

Additionally, both plain and herb-infused raw honey can be used topically in wound and burn healing. Its antimicrobial and antibacterial properties can support skin- and membrane-healing processes. It can also help fight stubborn antibiotic-resistant infections caused by staph bacteria.

Infused Oils

Infused oils are made of herbs whose essences are infused into an oil base. They can be used topically or mixed with beeswax

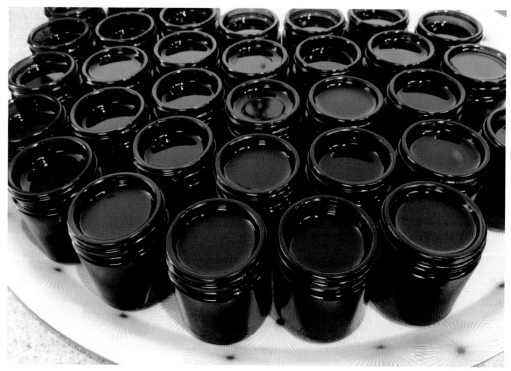
Jars filled with infused oil.

to create salves. (Note that oil-based preparations should not be applied to open wounds.) Infused oils can be made from fresh or dry plant material by heating or by letting the infusion sit in a sunny spot so that the plant's essences can transfer into the oil.

If you are working with fresh plants, it is important that you infuse the oils long enough with a consistent heat source to ensure that any potential moisture in the fresh plant material is evaporated to avoid the oil becoming rancid or spoiled.

The solar infusion technique uses the sun to prepare herbs. Place the herbs and oil in a sunny spot for several weeks until the infusion is complete. This is a good method if you live in an area with regular, consistent sun availability. Because I live in an area with inconsistent sunlight, I set up my slow-cooker to use as a bain-marie (or water bath).

The warm water helps extract the herbal essences into the oil, evaporate moisture from fresh plant materials, and mitigate the heat from the coil in the unit.

To make an herbal oil infusion in a slow-cooker, you'll need jars, herbs, and oil. Fill the jars with plant material and cover with oil. Then place the jars in the water-filled cooker, covered with cheesecloth. Set the cooker on warm. The oil in the jars should reach about 120°F.

Allow the jars to remain in the water bath for a few days or until the oil achieves the color, odor, and strength that you want. To test the oil's moisture level, place a glass lid over the jar. If water condenses under the lid, keep the jars in the warm bath to evaporate existing moisture in the oil.

Strain the finished oil and store it in jars for topical use, or use it to prepare an herbal salve.

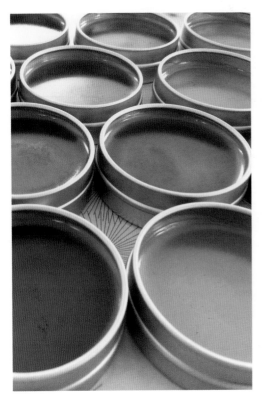

Tins of salve cool on the counter.

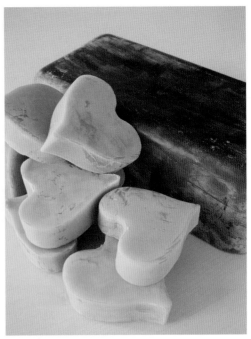

Every home herbalist should have beeswax on hand—particularly the local kind, which smells divine. Beeswax is a key ingredient in making salves, balms, and creams.

Salves

As we read more and more information regarding the toxicity of commercially available topical creams, cosmetics, and cleansers, making healthful skin preparations is an easy solution that avoids the chemicals—and it can save us a bit of money on beauty care. Blending infused oils with beeswax can also result in useful salves for the medicine kit.

Every home herbalist should have beeswax on hand—particularly the local kind, which smells divine. Beeswax is a key ingredient in making salves, balms, and creams.

Several medicinal plants are great for use in topical salves, including arnica, comfrey, dandelion flower, goldenrod, motherwort leaf, Solomon's seal, St. John's wort, violet leaf, and yarrow.

To create salve, you will need 8 ounces of herb-infused oil and 1 ounce of beeswax. Place the oil and beeswax in the top of a double-boiler and heat until the beeswax melts. Adjust the consistency by adding more wax or oil, depending on your preference. Remove the pan from heat, and pour the mixture into prepared tins or jars. A drop or two of vitamin E oil can help preserve the salve and extend its shelf life. Store the salve in a cool location; it should last a year or more. If the salve smells rancid, discontinue using it and discard it.

WILDCRAFTING FOR WELLNESS

A SEASON-BY-SEASON HARVEST GUIDE

The four seasons of the Midwest create a dynamic wildcrafting calendar for the herbalist. Tree barks are most easily gathered in the spring or fall, or in the summer after a wild storm, when the fallen branches rest on the forest floor. Fruiting shrubs and trees set flower in spring and then yield succulent berries, mostly sweet under the hot summer sun. Even beneath a quiet blanket of winter snow, the plants can yield an adventure in wildcrafting and offer medicine.

What follows is a simple outline that will help you learn the seasonal patterns of wild plants. The Midwest covers a great deal of territory and several climates—for example, the growing season in South Dakota is significantly shorter than the season in southern Ohio. A plant's bloom time in one part of the Midwest can be very different from its bloom time elsewhere. Other factors that can affect harvesting times include microclimates with varying elevation, soils, and weather (especially around the Great Lakes). Take these factors into consideration when creating your own wildcrafting calendar.

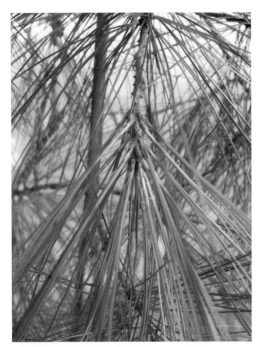

White pine is a perfect early spring plant to wildcraft and use to ward off colds that come with the season's change.

EARLY SPRING

As the snow melts from the fields and woodlands, the early greens of spring begin to emerge. Early spring is an excellent time to gather tree barks, twig tips, and small branches for making tea and other herbal remedies. The sap is still running through the trees, which makes the bark easier to process. Tubers, roots, and rhizomes may be gathered at this time, before the plants begin to move significant energy upward to grow stems, leaves, and flowers.

Where to Wildcraft Early Spring Plants

Full Sun: Open Fields, Disturbed Open Spaces, and Edges of the Woods

- agrimony flowers, leaves
- burdock roots
- butterfly weed roots
- catnip leaves
- ceanothus inner bark, roots
- chickweed flowers, leaves, stems
- comfrey leaves
- dandelion leaves, roots
- evening primrose leaves
- field garlic bulbs, leaves
- juniper leaves
- lemon balm leaves
- motherwort leaves
- mullein leaves, roots
- Oregon grape leaves, rhizomes
- ox-eye daisy leaves
- plantain leaves
- poke roots
- prickly ash bark
- prickly pear pads
- raspberry leaves, roots
- red clover leaves
- uva-ursi leaves

Wetlands, Riverbeds, and Lakesides

- alder inner and outer bark, leaves
- calamus leaves, rhizomes
- cottonwood buds, twigs
- crampbark bark, twigs
- nettle leaves
- peppermint flowers, leaves, stems
- yellow birch bark, leaf buds, leaves, sap, twigs

Woodlands and Partial Shade

- aspen inner and outer bark, twigs
- barberry bark, root bark
- black cherry inner bark
- blackberry leaves
- chaga fruiting body
- cleavers flowers, leaves, stems
- coltsfoot flowers, leaves, stalks
- dock leaves, roots
- eastern white cedar leaves
- lovage roots
- lungwort flowers, leaves
- oak bark, leaves

partridge berry leaves, stems
pine bark, needles, resin
pedicularis flowers, leaves
pipsissewa leaves
reishi fruiting body
sassafras leaves, roots
slippery elm inner bark
Solomon's seal rhizomes
spicebush leaves, twigs
spruce branch tips, shoots
tulip poplar branch tips
wild geranium roots
wild ginger rhizomes
wild yam rhizomes
wintergreen leaves

MID- TO LATE SPRING

In midspring, the temperature and soil begin to warm. Early spring plants send up flower stalks, and the summer perennials unfurl their first leaves. This is a perfect time to begin gathering tender leaves and flowers for teas, herbal remedies, and simple syrups.

Where to Wildcraft Mid- to Late Spring Plants

Full Sun: Open Fields, Disturbed Open Spaces, and Edges of the Woods

apple bark, flowers, leaves, twigs
artemisia leaves
borage flowers, leaves
burdock roots
catnip leaves
chickweed flowers, leaves, stems
comfrey flowers, leaves, stalks
dandelion flowers, leaves, roots
dock roots
echinacea aerial parts, roots
evening primrose flowers, leaves
ground ivy flowers, leaves, stems
hawthorn flowers, leaves, thorns
juniper leaves

lemon balm leaves, stems
motherwort leaves
mullein leaves
Oregon grape leaves
ox-eye daisy flowers, leaves
plantain leaves
poke roots
prickly ash bark
prickly pear pads
raspberry leaves, roots
red clover flowers, leaves
rose leaves, petals
shepherd's purse leaves, seedpods, stems
spotted bee balm leaves
uva-ursi leaves
violet flowers, leaves
wild bergamot leaves
wild peach flowers, leaves, young twigs

Wetlands, Riverbeds, and Lakesides

alder strobiles, twigs
angelica leaves
calamus rhizomes
horsetail aerial parts
peppermint flowers, leaves, stems
spearmint leaves

Woodlands and Partial Shade

blackberry leaves
black cherry flowers, inner bark, twigs
chaga fruiting body
cleavers flowers, leaves, stems
coltsfoot flowers, leaves
eastern white cedar leaves
jewelweed leaves, stems
oak bark, leaves
partridge berry leaves, stems
pine needles
pipsissewa leaves
reishi fruiting body
sassafras leaves, roots
skullcap flowers, leaves, stems
Solomon's seal rhizomes

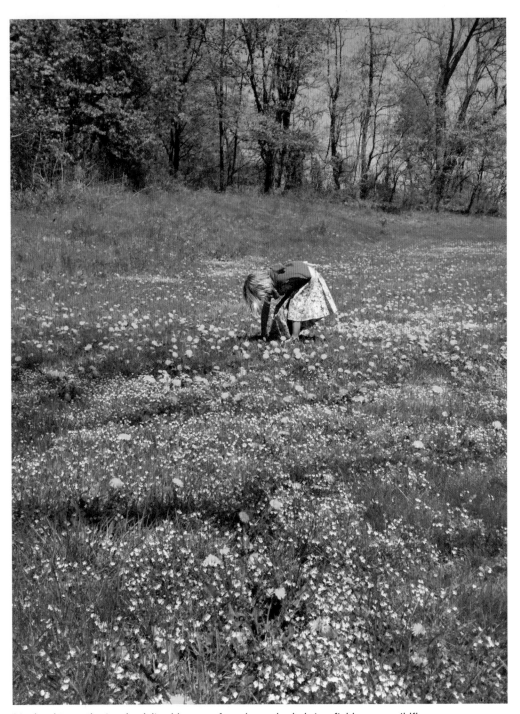

My daughter gathering dandelion blossoms for salve and salads in a field among wildflowers.

spicebush leaves, twigs
spruce needles
tulip poplar branch tips
turkey tail fruiting body
wild geranium leaves, roots
wild ginger rhizomes
wild yam rhizomes
wintergreen berries, leaves

SUMMER

Summer is a magical time in the woods and fields in the Midwest. The smell of sweet clover fills the air, crickets chirp, and in the evening lightning bugs fill the sky. Plant harvests are bountiful, especially with all of the aromatic flowers and medicinal berries to gather for teas and tinctures. This is the season for goldenrod, which can be used to create wonderful musculoskeletal plant medicines.

Where to Wildcraft Summer Plants

Full Sun: Open Fields, Disturbed
Open Spaces, and Edges of the Woods

catnip flowers
blue vervain flowers, leaves
boneset flowers
borage flowers, leaves
burdock roots
evening primrose flowers, leaves
feverfew flowers, leaves
goldenrod flowers, leaves
grindelia flowers, leaves
hawkweed aerial parts
honeysuckle flowers
horehound flowers, leaves, stems
hyssop flowers, leaves
Joe Pye weed aerial parts
Lemon balm flowers, leaves, stems
motherwort flowers
mullein flowers, leaves
Oregon grape leaves

pennycress seeds
plantain seeds
poke roots
prickly pear pads
raspberry fruit, leaves, roots
red clover flowers, leaves
rose leaves, petals
Russian sage flowers, leaves
shepherd's purse seedpods
spotted bee balm flowers, leaves
St. John's wort flowers, leaves
sweet clover flowers, leaves
uva-ursi leaves
valerian flowers, leaves
wild bergamot flowers, leaves
wild peach leaves
yarrow flowers, leaves

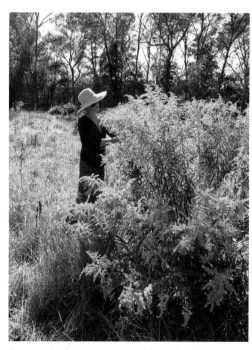

Summer is the season for goldenrod, which can be used to create wonderful musculoskeletal plant medicines.

Wetlands, Riverbeds, and Lakesides

- angelica leaves, roots, seeds
- elder berries, flowers
- horsetail aerial parts
- meadowsweet flowers
- peppermint flowers, leaves, stems
- spearmint flowers, leaves

Woodlands and Partial Shade

- arnica whole plant
- black cherry fruit
- black walnut hulls
- chaga fruiting body
- eastern white cedar leaves
- ghost pipe aerial parts
- jewelweed flowers, leaves, stems
- lady's mantle flowers, leaves, roots
- linden bracts, flowers
- lobelia flowers, leaves, seedpods
- lovage flowers, leaves, seeds
- oak bark, leaves
- partridge berry leaves, stems
- pine needles
- pipsissewa leaves
- reishi fruiting body
- sassafras leaves
- self-heal flowers, leaves
- skullcap flowers, leaves, stems
- Solomon's seal rhizomes
- spicebush berries, leaves, twigs
- tulip poplar branch tips, flowers
- wintergreen leaves
- wood betony flowers, leaves

FALL

Fall is a special harvest season for the medicine-maker. It's the time to dig up roots, tubers, and rhizomes to preserve in infused oils and tinctures and to collect the last of the summer's herbs and flowers before the frosts and snow arrive.

Where to Wildcraft Fall Plants

Full Sun: Open Fields, Disturbed Open Spaces, and Edges of the Woods

- apple fruit
- barberry bark, root bark
- burdock roots
- butterfly weed roots
- catnip leaves
- ceanothus roots
- chickweed leaves
- dandelion leaves, roots
- dock roots, seeds
- echinacea aerial parts, roots
- elecampane roots
- evening primrose roots
- ginkgo fruit, leaves
- goldenrod flowers, leaves
- hawthorn fruit
- Joe Pye weed roots
- juniper berries, leaves
- lemon balm leaves
- mullein leaves, roots
- New England aster flowers, leaves
- Oregon grape leaves, rhizomes
- plantain leaves
- poke roots
- prickly ash bark
- prickly pear fruit, pads
- raspberry leaves, roots
- red clover leaves
- rose hips, leaves
- Russian sage flowers, leaves
- spotted bee balm flowers, leaves
- uva-ursi leaves
- violet flowers, leaves
- wild bergamot flowers, leaves
- yarrow leaves

Wetlands, Riverbeds, and Lakesides

- angelica roots, seeds
- calamus rhizomes
- cranberry fruit

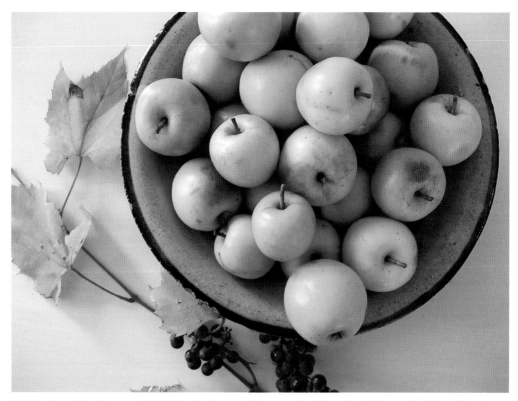

Wild apples bring the scent of fall. Their skins contain aromatic oils, acids, bitter and astringent tannins, yeasts, and pigments high in antioxidants.

horsetail aerial parts
nettle leaves, seeds
peppermint flowers, leaves, stems
spearmint leaves

Woodlands and Partial Shade

beechnuts
blackberry roots
chaga fruiting body
coltsfoot roots
eastern white cedar leaves
lobelia flowers, leaves, seedpods
maitake fruiting body
oak bark, leaves
partridge berry leaves, stems
pine needles
pipsissewa leaves
reishi fruiting body

sassafras leaves, roots
Solomon's seal rhizomes
spicebush berries, leaves, twigs
turkey tail fruiting body
wild geranium leaves, roots
wild ginger rhizomes
wild yam rhizomes
wintergreen leaves
witch hazel flowers, leaves, twigs

WINTER

Folks frequently ask, "Can you wildcraft in winter?" and my response is always a resounding "Yes!" Although there are no summer berries and flowers to be found in the deep snow of the Midwest, an herbalist can delight in wildcrafting barks, buds, and even sap in the coldest winter months.

Not only can many plants be gathered in the winter, but wintertime is a perfect chance to hone your plant identification skills. Practice keying out plants and trees from last season's leaves, stalks, and barks and discover new plant stands for spring harvesting.

I firmly believe that we should spend time outdoors in all four seasons. It helps with seasonal depression, it can boost immunity, and it's good for the soul to get outside and appreciate the natural world around us.

Where to Wildcraft Winter Plants

Full Sun: Open Fields, Disturbed Open Spaces, and Edges of the Woods

juniper berries, leaves
poke roots
uva-ursi leaves

Wetlands, Riverbeds, and Lakesides

cottonwood buds
cranberry fruit
yellow birch sap

Woodlands and Partial Shade

beech ghost leaves
reishi fruiting body
spicebush berries, leaves, twigs
wintergreen leaves

WILD MEDICINAL PLANTS OF THE MIDWEST

Blue vervain

agrimony

Agrimonia species

PARTS USED flowers, leaves

This small and unassuming perennial is used as a relaxant in formulas to ease many modern ailments, including excess mental tension resulting from overachieving.

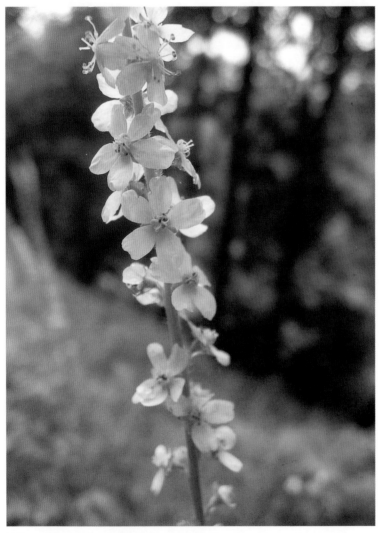

Yellow agrimony flowers grow on slender spikes. Combine agrimony with blue vervain to help calm the mind and relieve anxiety and mental tension.

How to Identify

Agrimony grows 12–24 inches tall, with dark green, deeply toothed foliage that is oblong, soft, and hairy. The pinnately compound leaves comprise six to nine major leaflets, with minor leaflets between them and a single terminal leaflet.

Agrimony flowers in early summer with several slender, leafless spikes of yellow blossoms, each with five oblong petals. The entire plant, including the root, has a pleasant floral odor. Before flowering, the entire plant tastes mildly sweet and sour. After flowering, it is more astringent tasting. In the fall, the flowers give way to small, sticky burs that contain seeds.

Where, When, and How to Wildcraft

Look for agrimony growing in sunny spots along the edges of the woods, in sun-dappled fields, or alongside hedgerows or woodland trails in dappled sunshine. Strip the leaves from the stems in the spring when they are young, before the plant flowers in early summer. Pick the flowers off the spike to use fresh or to dry for later use.

Medicinal Uses

Use fresh or dry leaves and flowers to prepare a tea or tincture that can help relieve muscle spasms and tension in the body, particularly with stomach pain or kidney stones. Mix agrimony with other herbs, such as St. John's wort and wild yam, to use as a pain reliever.

To ease tension associated with a type-A personality, combine agrimony with blue vervain to help calm the mind and relieve anxiety and mental tension. Use fresh flowers to prepare a flower essence in brandy.

Future Harvests

Harvest leaves and flowers from only a few stems from each plant to ensure plant sustainability.

HERBAL PREPARATIONS

Agrimony leaf tea
Infusion
Drink ¼ cup as needed.

Agrimony tincture
1 part fresh flowers and leaves
2 parts menstruum (50 percent alcohol, 50 percent distilled water)
or
1 part dry flowers and leaves
5 parts menstruum (50 percent alcohol, 50 percent distilled water)
Take 10–15 drops as needed.

alder

Alnus species

PARTS USED inner and outer bark, leaves, strobiles, twigs

As a lymphatic herb, alder helps restore proper digestion and provides support for the lymphatic system. For stagnation or sluggish digestion, alder can help return digestive processes back to normal.

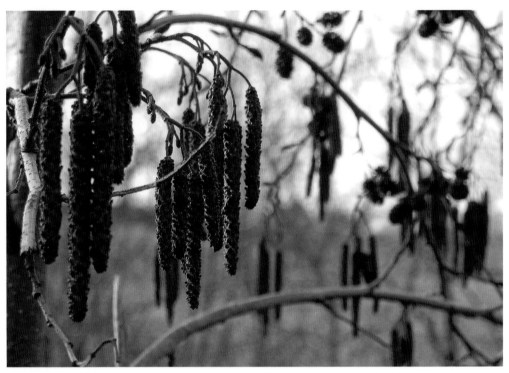

Alder strobiles are conelike, seed-bearing structures that hang from the branches.

How to Identify

Alder is a deciduous tree or shrub that grows in wetland areas and bogs and along stream banks. It grows in thickets as a shrub but can reach 20 feet tall or more when mature.

Alder bark is smooth and gray, and depending on the species, it can be furrowed or mottled with a green tinge. Alder leaves alternate on the branches and are small, egg-shaped, simple, and serrated.

In the winter, both male and shorter female strobiles emerge. Alder strobiles are notably bitter in flavor, but they are edible and can be used medicinally. Twigs and branches have a slightly sweet and bitter flavor, similar to that of birch or wild cherry wood, but less aromatic.

Where, When, and How to Wildcraft

Look for alders growing in any type of soil along stream banks and in wetland areas, or growing among conifers in a forest. In early spring, wildcraft the strobiles along with young twigs and branches. Wildcraft leaves as they unfurl in the spring, and peel the inner and outer bark from freshly felled branches after a spring windstorm.

Medicinal Uses

Use the bark, leaves, strobiles, and twigs fresh or dry them for later use. All parts can be blended and prepared as tincture or tea.

Consider alder to help with stagnation or sluggish digestion. If used regularly, it helps restore digestive processes and can be used with other metabolic tonifying herbs such as burdock root, yellow dock, or a carminative (gas-relieving) herb such as angelica to help strengthen the digestion.

For topical infections, prepare the bark, leaves, strobiles, and twigs as a decoction to use as a skin wash. Combine alder with echinacea for a good astringent and antiseptic skin-healing combination.

Lymphatics are also useful in treating musculoskeletal issues such as bursitis or rheumatic joint inflammation with excess fluid. Use alder tincture topically as a liniment for massage in combination with other musculoskeletal herbs such as goldenrod and mullein to help stimulate blood circulation and disperse the excess fluid in the inflamed area.

Future Harvests

Alder is prolific and invasive in some areas. The bark, leaves, strobiles, and twigs of the tree can be harvested without imposing significant harm. For sustainability, gather bark from fallen branches in lieu of harvesting it from live trees.

HERBAL PREPARATIONS

Alder tea
Decoction
Drink ¼ cup, or use externally as a topical wash.

Alder tincture
1 part fresh bark, leaves, strobiles, and twigs, chopped
2 parts menstruum (95 percent alcohol, 5 percent distilled water)
or
1 part dry bark, leaves, strobiles, and twigs, chopped
5 parts menstruum (95 percent alcohol, 5 percent distilled water)
Take 30 drops, 3 to 5 times per day, or use topically as a liniment.

angelica

Angelica atropurpurea

PARTS USED flowers, leaves, roots, seeds, stems

Angelica is a spicy, aromatic, and warming herb that can help ward off a chill that comes with a cold or flu, soothe an upset stomach, or warm a disheartened spirit with its delightful aromas.

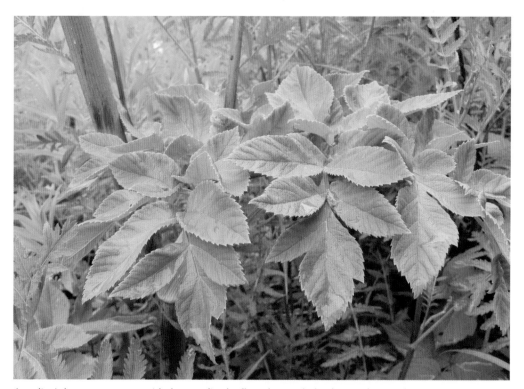

Angelica's leaves are ovate, with three to five leaflets that each divide into three to five segments.

How to Identify

Angelica is a member of the family Apiaceae—some of whose members, particularly poison hemlock (*Conium maculatum*), are deadly to humans and animals. It's important that you distinguish angelica from the poisonous plants in the family to avoid deadly accidents.

The stalk of angelica is hollow, smooth, and purple. Leaves are ovate, with three to five leaflets that divide further into three to five segments on each leaflet. Although angelica and poison hemlock stems can both show purple coloring, angelica stems tend to be uniformly purple, while poison hemlock's green stems are spotted or streaked with purple.

Angelica blossoms are white to yellow-green, arranged in globe-shaped, doubly-compound terminal clusters 2 to 6 inches

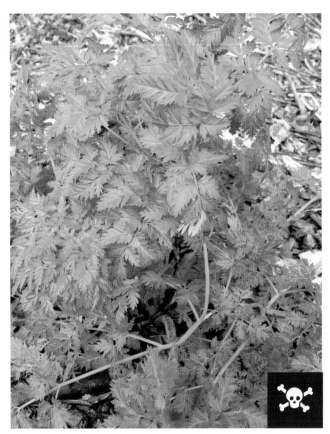

Poison hemlock leaves are more fernlike, green, and shiny than angelica leaves.

stands and tolerates shade well.

You can use the entire angelica plant, from roots to seeds. Harvest leaves in spring and summer and flowers in midsummer. Strip the leaves from the stem and dry them for tea.

It is easiest to harvest seeds and roots in dry weather in late summer or early fall, when the plant matures and seeds are dry, fully ripe, and ready for wildcrafting. Roots can be dug, washed, and dried for later use. At home, take time to ensure that seeds are dry and free of insects before storing them in an airtight container.

The bitter and aromatic flavors of angelica are similar to those of its super-herb cousin, osha (*Ligusticum porteri*); the impressions of the flavors— warming and drying—are less strong than that of osha but equally notable.

wide. (Poison hemlock's small white flowers grow in umbrella-shaped clusters.) Angelica produces creamy white and beige, broad, oval seeds. The entire plant, including the white and gnarled roots, smells strongly of celery, which is a chief identifier of angelica.

Angelica shows its first leaves in the early spring and flowers in midsummer, and it goes to seed and dies back in the late summer and early fall.

Where, When, and How to Wildcraft

Angelica grows in hedgerows and along the edges of the woods, usually in damp soil. Look for it in ravines, floodplains, ditches, and gullies. It can self-sow to create large

Medicinal Uses

Use fresh or dry roots and leaves to make a warming, aromatic tea, flavored with other herbs such as hyssop and sweetened with honey. Savor the tea to relieve a chill from cold, damp weather.

Angelica can also support a fever during a cold or the flu and can be added to blends of elderflower, mint, and yarrow to boost the body's immune system response to a viral infection. As an aromatic, angelica can soothe a stomachache or damp cough. A tincture of fresh or dry roots, leaves, and seeds can also help.

Nibble the seeds after a meal as a digestive aid, or chew them when you feel a cold coming

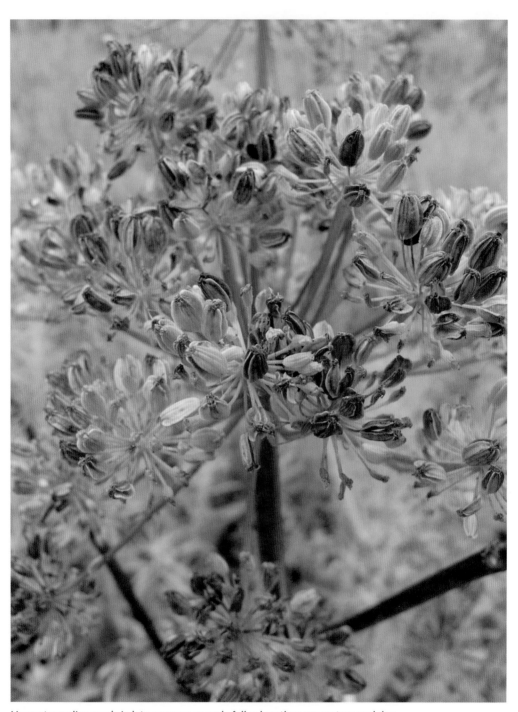

Harvest angelica seeds in late summer or early fall, when they are mature and dry.

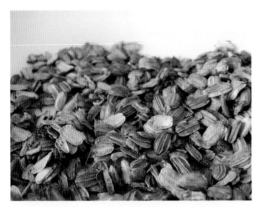

Angelica seeds are warming and aromatic in flavor. Chew them when you feel a cold coming on.

on. Use an alcohol-based root extraction to create an excellent cocktail cart staple.

Chop the fresh stalks and candy them using cane sugar for use in confections similar to candied ginger, or eat them alone as a treat. Offer them as a carminative herb to soothe a stomachache.

Angelica can help soothe a tired and worn spirit resulting from heartache and sadness. Chew the seeds, or add the leaves to a blend with hawthorn or rose to make a soothing tea to ease grief.

Future Harvests

Although angelica can self-sow and spread rapidly in favorable conditions, consider the impact on the size of the plantings of angelica if you are harvesting the plant for its roots. If you are harvesting a large quantity and are concerned about the population in the area, you can propagate angelica from cuttings.

 Cautions, Concerns, and Considerations

If you have any doubt about the plant's identification, do not crush it with your fingers to smell it unless you are wearing gloves, because the toxicity of poison hemlock can be absorbed through the skin simply by handling the plant. Certainly do not taste the plant if you are unsure of its identity.

Seek an experienced plant medicine-maker or botanist who can help you confirm the plant's identification and safety. Once you do learn its chief characteristics and can safely identify it, angelica is a valuable addition to the apothecary and the spice cabinet.

HERBAL PREPARATIONS

Angelica tea
Infusion
Drink ¼ cup as needed.

Angelica tincture
1 part fresh flowers, leaves, roots, seeds, and stems, chopped
2 parts menstruum (50 percent alcohol, 50 percent distilled water)
or
1 part dry flowers, leaves, roots, seeds, and stems, chopped
4 parts menstruum (50 percent alcohol, 50 percent distilled water)
Take 10–15 drops in water, as needed.

---

apple

Malus species
PARTS USED bark, flowers, fruit, leaves, twigs

An apple a day keeps the doctor away. You can rely on wild apple as a valued plant for the kitchen and apothecary, where its bark, flowers, fruit, leaves, and twigs can be used on the dinner table or as medicine.

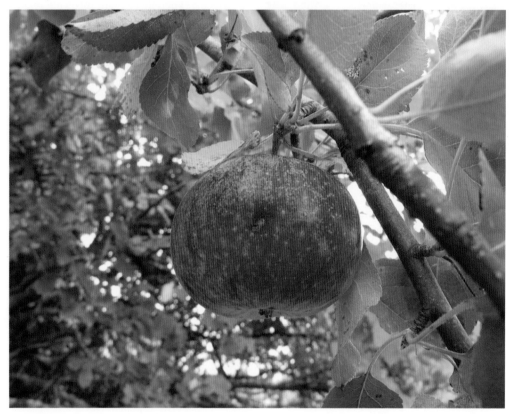

As an apple ripens, its color and aroma become more pronounced. The fruit can help soothe an upset digestive system.

How to Identify

This small fruiting tree has brown, scaly bark and dense branches. Its leaves are ovate with serrated margins and light-colored undersides. The five-petaled, pinkish to white flowers are arranged in corymbs, flat-topped clusters in which individual flower stalks grow from various points of the stem to reach the same height. The fragrant blossoms attract many honey bees throughout the spring.

The fruit of the wild apple grows in a range of colors—from yellow, to green, to red—and a broad range of flavors, including sweet, bitter, acidic, and sour. All are delicious.

Where, When, and How to Wildcraft

Wild apple trees grow across the Midwest in fields and hedgerows, on public lands, and near hiking trails. Apple trees are also common as ornamentals in urban landscapes, though many suburbanites and municipalities view the excess fruit as bothersome as it ripens and falls from the trees.

In late spring, wildcraft the blossoms and dry them for tincture or tea, or prepare them as flower essences. Carefully select a blossom or two from each corymb and collect the fragile blooms in a container, making sure they aren't crushed.

Wildcraft the fresh, green bark of twigs and the new leaves at the same time, using pruning shears to trim off the tips of the new growth and wildcrafting the leaves by hand.

Fruits ripen from mid- to late fall. An unripe apple's skin will be noticeably tannic, or tart, in flavor. As it ripens, it becomes more sweet and fragrant. Allow the apples to ripen fully and wildcraft the fallen fruit to ensure that you have gathered the sweetest and most aromatic fruit. Ripe apples detach easily from the tree, and freshly fallen apples are ripest. Look for apples that are free of insect damage; the fruit is frequently inhabited by moth larvae.

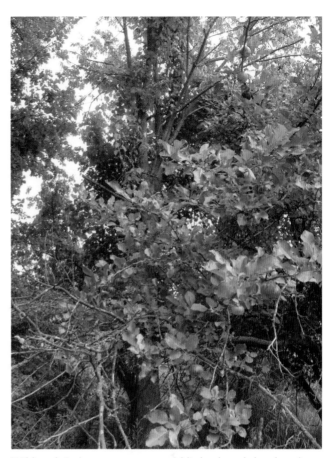

Wild apple trees are common on public lands and abandoned farmsteads in the fruit belt of the Midwest.

Medicinal Uses

A member of the rose family (Rosaceae), the apple is cooling and astringent when used medicinally. Prepare the blossoms and twigs fresh or dry them to use in astringent teas or topical washes. Use the tea as an astringent wash for weepy and drippy rashes such as poison ivy. Add chamomile and rose petals for their extra drying and soothing properties. Include blackberry root in tea to help soothe diarrhea.

The fruit can help soothe an upset digestive system; it can settle a stomach and help the body recover from vomiting, diarrhea, or food poisoning. Apple juice is also very nutritive for a debilitated or recovering digestive system.

Use wild apples to create a fine homemade raw apple cider vinegar, a valuable ingredient

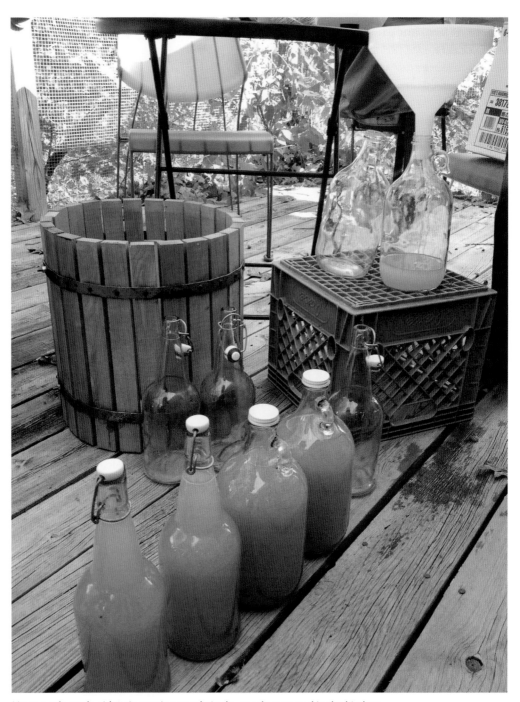

Homemade apple cider vinegar is a staple in the apothecary and in the kitchen.

for the herbalist's apothecary. Apple cider vinegar can be used as a menstruum for vinegar-based tinctures to extract minerals from plants and as a base for preparing fermented foods. Sweeten the cider with wild sugars such as raw honey.

Future Harvests

Wind-fallen wild apples are always in abundance, and wildcrafting them does not affect future harvests.

HERBAL PREPARATIONS

Apple blossom and twig tea
Infusion
Drink 1 cup as needed, or use externally as topical wash.

Apple tincture
1 part fresh leaves, twigs, and/or flowers, chopped
2 parts menstruum (50 percent alcohol, 50 percent distilled water)
or
1 part dry leaves, twigs, and/or flowers, chopped
4 parts menstruum (50 percent alcohol, 50 percent distilled water)
Take 15–25 drops as needed.

arnica

Arnica montana
PARTS USED whole plant

Life guarantees bumps and bruises, and arnica is a woodland plant favored by herbalists to help soothe the soreness and smooth out the pain. This herb promotes lymphatic flow and encourages circulation to an injured area.

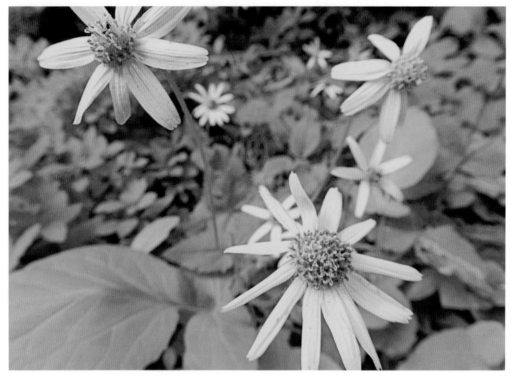

Arnica is useful for many musculoskeletal injuries, particularly sprains or bruises resulting from a trauma or blow.

How to Identify

Arnica is a hardy perennial that grows 12–24 inches tall, with oblong green leaves that grow in an opposite arrangement along the stem. In mid- to late summer, yellow daisylike flowers bloom with 12–14 petals, each about 1 inch long, with yellow to orange centers. The entire plant has a notably dry texture and is slightly aromatic with a bitter taste.

Where, When, and How to Wildcraft

Look for arnica in woodland areas with dappled shade at middle to high altitudes. Wildcraft the whole plant in summer at the beginning of its bloom time to ensure that you gather fresh, healthy plants.

Remove the roots, wash and chop them, and then use them fresh or dry them for later use. To dry the aerial parts, bundle and hang the stems. Dried blossoms are fluffy and fibrous.

Medicinal Uses

Arnica is indicated for many musculoskeletal injuries, particularly sprains and bruises. Fresh or dry plant materials can be prepared as tea for a topical compress or as a topical tincture to use as liniment. The entire plant can also be prepared as an herb-infused oil or salve to massage over an injured area.

Herbs that work well with arnica to help dispel bruising include calendula, goldenrod, mullein, and yarrow. To work with sharp shooting pain, combine arnica with St. John's wort. For achy pain, combine arnica with black cohosh and perhaps a warming herb such as cayenne or turmeric to help stimulate circulation to the area. For soft tissue injuries and joint pain, add Solomon's seal to help with healing.

Future Harvests

Although arnica is neither rare nor endangered, it is not widely distributed throughout the Midwest. Wildcraft only a few plants from each stand. Arnica also makes a great landscape plant to include in a permaculture design plan for a home herb garden.

HERBAL PREPARATIONS

Arnica tea
Decoction
Use externally as a topical wash or muscle compress.

Arnica tincture
1 part fresh flowers, leaves, roots, and
   stems, chopped
2 parts menstruum (50 percent alcohol,
   50 percent distilled water)
or
1 part dry flowers, leaves, roots, and stems,
   chopped
4 parts menstruum (50 percent alcohol,
   50 percent distilled water)
Take 10–15 drops internally, or use topically as a liniment, diluted with equal parts water.

Arnica-infused oil
1 part fresh flowers, leaves, roots, and
   stems, chopped
2 parts oil
or
1 part dry flowers, leaves, roots, and stems,
   chopped
4 parts oil
Use for massage.

artemisia

Artemisia species

mugwort, wormwood

PARTS USED leaves

With a rich plant lore and a variety of medicinal uses for digestive distress and fever, artemisia holds an important place in the herbal apothecary.

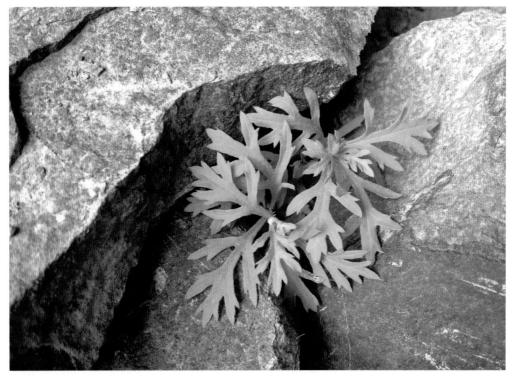

The silvery leaves of artemisia are used in medicinal teas and tinctures. Look for artemisia in rocky, craggy outcrops and disturbed areas where it grows in hot, dry soil in full sun.

How to Identify

Artemisia is an herbaceous perennial genus that comprises about 180 species. Plants grow to about 4 feet tall and 2½ feet wide at maturity. Smooth, silvery, lobed leaves are 2–3 inches long and arranged in a spiral on woody stems. Clusters of yellow flower heads emerge from the leaf axils from midsummer to early fall.

Where, When, and How to Wildcraft

Look for artemisia in rocky, craggy outcrops and disturbed areas, where it grows in hot, dry soil in full sun.

The plant's new growth in early spring is more fragrant than bitter, especially before flowering. Wildcraft the leaves in the spring before plants begin to flower to ensure the best aromatic qualities. Prepare the leaves fresh or dry and store them in an airtight container for later use.

Medicinal Uses

A staple in the herbal apothecary, this astringent herb is a must-have for settling a turbulent upset stomach. The bitters of artemisia are cold and drying. When made into tincture, artemisia is helpful to use for digestive distress or as a stomach tonic in the event of a virus or intestinal bacterial infection.

A tincture of *Artemisia absinthium* or *A. vulgaris* should be included in the traveler's first aid kit to be used to ward off the ill effects of traveler's tummy or an unexpected case of the stomach flu.

For fevers, artemisia can help support the body's natural processes of fighting illness, as a diaphoretic that helps the body produce sweat. A hot artemisia tea, while markedly bitter in taste, can help facilitate this and combines well with the relaxant properties of elderflower and mint. A cold infusion of artemisia can help temper the bitterness, especially when it's sweetened with honey.

Artemisia-infused vodka can serve as a base for simple cocktail bitters—good on its own or blended with other flavors, including citrus and dark rum. Or consider adding a warming spice such as cardamom, cinnamon, orange zest, or spicebush. Use artemisia to flavor honey meads or homemade walnut nocino liqueur.

Included in a medicine bundle, artemisia can be used as a talisman to facilitate dream states or ward off the evil eye.

Future Harvests

Artemisia is a wild-growing perennial herb that can also be included in the herbalist's garden space. Wildcrafting its new growth will not affect the plant and can actually help encourage new shoots.

HERBAL PREPARATIONS

Artemisia absinthium leaf tea
Cold infusion
Drink ⅛ cup as needed.

Artemisia tridentata leaf tea
Cold infusion
Drink ⅛ cup as needed.

Artemisia vulgaris leaf tea
Hot infusion
Drink ¼ cup as needed.

Artemisia tincture
1 part dry *A. vulgaris* or *A. absinthium* leaves, chopped
5 parts menstruum (50 percent alcohol, 50 percent distilled water)
Take 10-25 drops as needed.

aspen

Populus tremuloides
quaking aspen
PARTS USED inner and outer bark, twigs

Aspen bark has a complex flavor that is perfect for delicious herbal bitters or for an aromatic tea that soothes digestion.

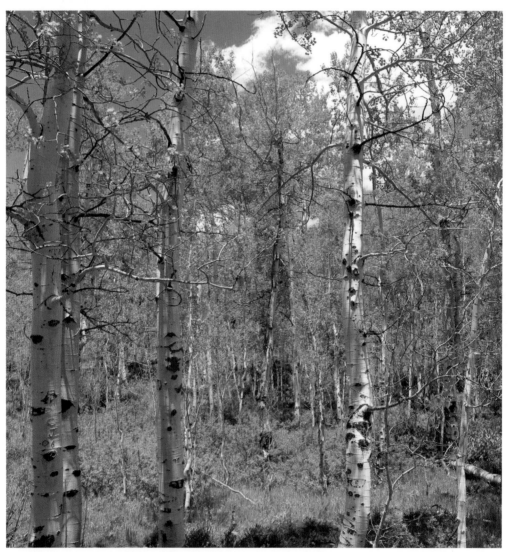

Use aspen bark to create delicious digestive bitters. The vanilla notes of the bark pair well with the flavors of angelica, blackberry, and maple syrup.

Selecting and Processing Tree Bark

Tree bark is a staple of plant medicine-makers. We wildcraft aspen, cherry, and yellow birch bark as well as bark of crampbark, oak, slippery elm, willow, and witch hazel, among others, for our herbal apothecaries.

Wildcrafting and stripping bark is fairly straightforward, but keep in mind that bark is easiest to wildcraft in the early spring, when the sap flows through the tree, making the outer and inner barks easier to peel away from the inner cambium layer.

Trees grow with a protective outer bark and an inner bark. For most medicinal preparations, you should wildcraft the inner bark. To access the inner bark, first peel the outer bark vertically off the wood in long, narrow strips. Then pull and scrape the inner bark away from the outer bark (methods will vary from tree-to-tree). Once removed, the inner bark can be used fresh, or dry it for later use. Store it completely dry in a sealed container.

In early spring, I frequently clip the new, young twigs and branch tips from live aspen, cherry, crampbark, tulip poplar, and yellow birch trees to make extracts and teas. I taste and chew the tips to get a sense of their flavor. If the tips are aromatic, I can process the twigs and tips into plant extracts or dry them and store them to use later.

How to Identify

The bark of young aspens is notably smooth and greenish gray or white. Silver dollar–sized leaves are triangular or heart-shaped, and they quake, or rustle, in the slightest breeze because of their flattened leafstalks. In the fall, leaves turn bright yellow; a shimmering aspen stand against a blue autumn sky is a sight to remember.

Where, When, and How to Wildcraft

Look for stands of aspen growing along stream banks and at the edges of meadows. Aspens are also common in dry woods at higher elevations.

Harvest aspen bark in the early spring by pruning twigs and branch tips from young saplings. Use your sense of smell and taste by chewing on a twig to discern its aromatics and bitterness.

Medicinal Uses

Use aspen bark to create delicious digestive bitters. The vanilla notes of the bark pair well with the flavors of angelica, blackberry, and maple syrup. Use the bitters to soothe digestive upsets or to flavor a rum-based cocktail.

Process the twigs and inner bark into tincture, or dry them on a screen and store them in a container when completely dry for later use. Use the aromatic alcohol extract of aspen bark in place of almond extract to lend a wild note to your baking projects.

Aspen bark tea is aromatic and bitter, with a back note of almond flavor. It blends well with acorn hulls, sarsaparilla, sassafras, spicebush, and wild ginger leaves for a wildcrafted chai tea. This warming, spicy tea can soothe a chill or ease indigestion caused by overindulgence. Or simply enjoy its full flavor on a crisp fall day.

Future Harvests

If you are wildcrafting small batches of bark for home use, you should not need to harvest these from living trees. Instead, seek out freshly cut trees or freshly fallen branches after a spring storm. Or, because home

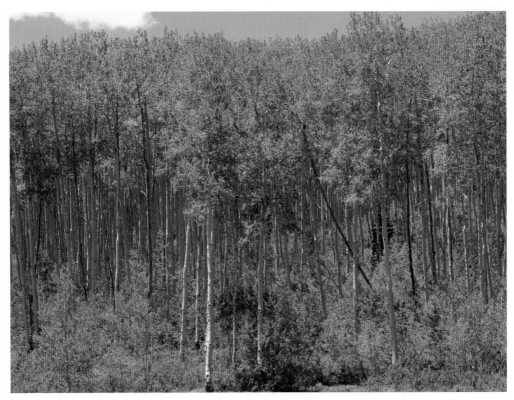

Aspen trees grow in large stands, interconnected to other trees by a complex underground root system.

garden tree pruning is often done in early spring, contact a local tree service and ask for branches of the specific tree you're looking for. If you do harvest from a living tree, be mindful and never remove the bark all the way around the trunk; this will kill the tree.

HERBAL PREPARATIONS

Aspen bark tea
Decoction
Drink ¼ cup.

Aspen tincture
1 part fresh bark and twigs, chopped
2 parts menstruum (95 percent alcohol,
   5 percent distilled water)
or
1 part dry bark and twigs, chopped
5 parts menstruum (95 percent alcohol,
   5 percent distilled water)
Take 10–15 drops as needed.

barberry

Berberis species
PARTS USED bark, root bark

With its powerful antibacterial and antibiotic properties, barberry is helpful in wound care as a remedy to protect against infection.

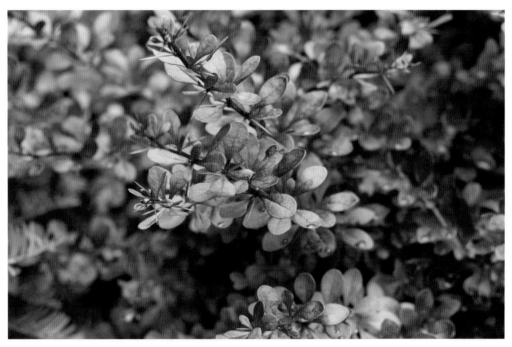

The berberine content in barberry makes it useful as an alternative to goldenseal, which has become endangered because of overharvesting.

How to Identify

This branched, woody shrub with gray bark can reach 10 feet tall at maturity. Primary and secondary leaves grow alternately on woody, branched shoots with sharp spines.

Barberry flowers in early summer with yellow panicles, or clusters, of flowers that hang below the branches. Its small red berries resemble cranberries in color, size (½ inch long), and tartness, and they are easily recognizable in winter. Both the soft bark and roots of the barberry are distinctly yellow, which is attributed to the berberine (an alkaloid plant extract) in the plant. This is the same chemical constituent that gives goldenseal its yellow color. Barberry is similar to goldenseal in astringency and bitterness.

Where, When, and How to Wildcraft

Look for barberry in dry woods and at the edges of the woods, in fields, or in open and disturbed waste places. Barberry is also grown as an ornamental in many urban gardens. Wildcraft the bark in early spring or late fall. Slice it into strips to use fresh, or dry it for later use.

Medicinal Uses

Prepare barberry bark as a tea or decoction to use as a wash for topical wounds, or prepare it as a tincture to take internally for infection. Both the tea and tincture can be diluted in a nasal saline wash to help clear sinus infections. Its bitterness is also helpful in stimulating stagnant digestion.

The berberine content in the barberry makes it useful as an alternative to goldenseal, which has become endangered because of overharvesting.

Future Harvests

Barberry grows abundantly across the Midwest. Wildcrafting the bark and roots from larger stands will not significantly impact the plant's distribution.

HERBAL PREPARATIONS

Barberry tea
Decoction
Drink ¼ cup as needed, or use externally as a topical or saline wash.

Barberry tincture
1 part fresh bark and root bark, chopped
2 parts menstruum (50 percent alcohol, 50 percent distilled water)
or
1 part dry bark and root bark, chopped
4 parts menstruum (50 percent alcohol, 50 percent distilled water)
Take 25–30 drops as needed, or use externally as a topical wash after diluting with equal parts water.

beech

Fagus grandifolia
PARTS USED leaves, nuts

Use beechnuts to make a nourishing chai tea. Its dry ghost leaves are useful in creating an astringent field medicine to clean mucosa and care for wounds.

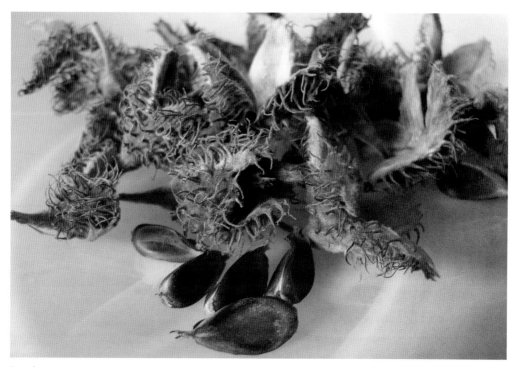

Beechnuts are nestled inside prickly husks. Crush and boil the nuts and hulls to make a mineral-rich, nutty drink.

How to Identify

The American beech can reach a height of 120 feet, with a diameter of 4–5 feet at maturity. The smooth bark is a steely, blue-gray color. The vibrant green and shiny leaves are 2–5 inches long and ovate, serrated, and slightly toothed. They change to an opaque cream color in winter—some call them ghost leaves—and stay on the branches long into the cold season, which makes the tree easy to identify at this time of year. A pair of three-sided nuts are usually held inside each prickly four-sided husk that falls from the tree in mid- to late fall.

Where, When, and How to Wildcraft

Beech is most common in mixed hardwood forests, often growing with maple and oak trees in rich, well-drained soil. When the beech matures, at about 40 years old, it begins to produce nut crops in the mid- to late fall, every three to five years. Your

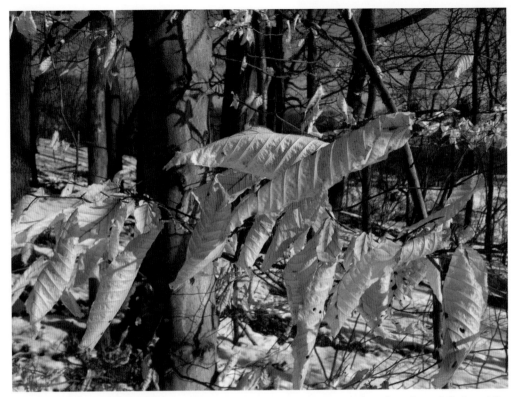

Dry ghost leaves remain attached to the tree in fall and winter. For a topical wash, make an infusion of the dry leaves.

competition for wildcrafting will be local wildlife, many of which enjoy beechnuts. So when the nuts begin to fall, you need to work fast to beat the rush. Harvest the ghost leaves from the tree in the late fall and winter.

Medicinal Uses

Crush and boil the nuts and hulls to make a mineral-rich, nutty drink, and consider blending the beechnut beverage into a local nut chai or hot cocoa with hickory nuts.

For a topical wash, make an infusion of the dry leaves. Strain and use this topically to clean and astringe weepy wounds. Or use it as an eyewash to clean the eye of debris or as part of a protocol for healing conjunctivitis (consider blending in chamomile for this use).

Future Harvests

Gathering nuts and ghost leaves from the beech will not affect future harvests. Tree plantings and preserving mixed hardwood habitats are important to the future of the American beech.

HERBAL PREPARATIONS

Beech hull and nutmeat tea
Decoction
Drink 1 cup as needed.

Beech ghost leaf tea
Infusion
Strain and use externally to flush debris from the eye, or use as an astringent wound wash.

blackberry

Rubus species

PARTS USED berries, leaves, roots

The delicious blackberry, known for its yummy summer berries, is also a useful medicinal plant. It offers mineral-dense leaves for nourishing infusions and astringent roots useful for stomach ailments.

How to Identify

Blackberries usually grow in sandy, well-drained soils, in large brambles along the sunny edges of woodlands. Growing to 13 feet long, blackberry canes are covered in thorns, with divided leaf clusters of three to five serrated and ovate leaflets with a prickly midrib. The blackberry blooms in late spring with five-petaled white flowers that bear seedy, slightly hairy fruit that ripens into dark purple berries in late summer.

Where, When, and How to Wildcraft

Look for blackberry brambles growing at the edges of woodlands, in vacant urban lots, and at roadsides. In the early spring, before the blackberry blooms, wildcraft leaves using a pair of scissors and carefully (being mindful of the thorns) clip off the leaf clusters to dry for use in tea. Pick the berries in late summer.

If you plan to harvest the roots, wait until fall when the plant begins to die back. Use a shovel and pruners. The roots are quite spindly, so a considerable amount of them are needed for a well-stocked apothecary. Wash, chop, and dry them for tea.

Medicinal Uses

Use blackberry leaves to create a mineral-dense, nourishing decoction. The leaves are high in calcium, iron, phosphorus, potassium, and zinc, as well as vitamins A, B, C,

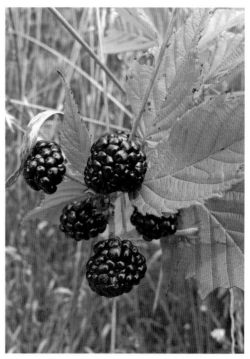

Blackberries are delicious, and the plant's leaves can be decocted for a mineral-dense, nourishing infusion.

and E. Extract the minerals by boiling the leaves for 20 minutes and enjoy them in a strong hot or iced tea. Blackberry leaves mix well with nettle, oatstraw, and red clover for a nutritious drink. If it tastes too earthy, add ice to mellow the mineral flavor a bit. Aromatics such as spicebush or the bark of aspen, birch, or tulip poplar can be added to spice up the tea, if preferred.

Prepared as an astringent tea, blackberry roots are used as a traditional remedy for diarrhea. Blend the roots with cocoa or chai to help settle and dry up the condition and soothe the stomach. Add honey to sweeten.

Future Harvests

Blackberries spread easily by runners, and the plant medicine-maker can encourage this process by cultivating runners in the immediate area to grow the stand, if necessary. Wildlife enjoy eating blackberries, and this should be a harvesting consideration, though wildcrafting the berries shouldn't significantly impact the production. Because blackberries grow prolifically, harvesting a few roots won't impact the plants, but if there is a concern, use leaves instead of roots to create tea.

Cautions, Concerns, and Considerations

Before harvesting wild berries, make sure the area has not been sprayed with herbicides, and get permission from the property owner when the vines grow on private land.

HERBAL PREPARATIONS

Blackberry leaf tea
Decoction
Drink 1–3 cups per day, or use as an astringent topical wash.

Blackberry root tea
Decoction
Drink 1 cup as needed, or use as an astringent topical wash.

Prunus serotina

PARTS USED bark, flowers, fruit, twigs

Black cherry bark is known by many herbalists as a relaxant cough remedy, but the flowers and twigs can also be used to flavor elixirs, as digestive bitters, and in cooking. Use the fruit juice in a healthful antioxidant drink.

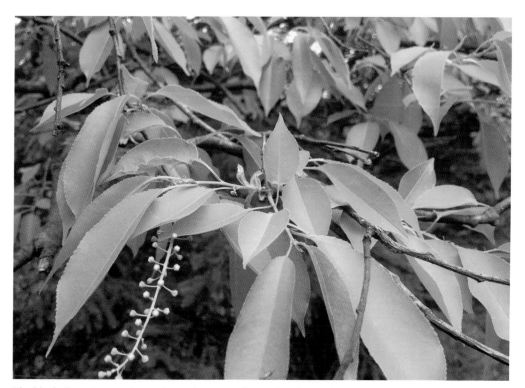

The black cherry's green leaves have shiny topsides, and underneath each there may be a slightly hairy midrib near the stem. Wildcraft young twigs for a cherry bark extract and collect flowers for a tincture or infusion.

How to Identify

A mature black cherry tree can grow upwards of 100 feet. The bark of a young tree is a steely dark gray, nearly black, and scored with horizontal lenticels, or pores. As the tree matures, its bark becomes rough and shaggy and is often said to resemble a burnt potato chip.

Its dark green leaves have shiny topsides, and underneath each, at least early in the season, there may be a slightly hairy midrib near the stem. Leaves are arranged alternately and are narrow and lanceolate with serrated edges.

Small white flowers in long racemes burst into bloom in late April and early May,

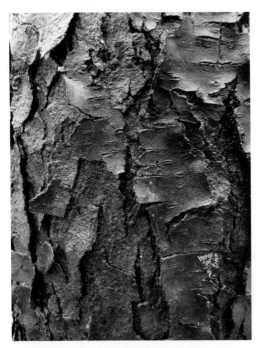

As the black cherry tree matures, the bark becomes rough and shaggy, often characterized as looking like a burnt potato chip.

making black cherry one of the earliest flowering wild fruit trees. Fruits are smaller than cultivated cherries and ripen in late summer in clusters of up to two-dozen pea-sized cherries that are bitter and somewhat sweet in flavor.

Where, When, and How to Wildcraft

Black cherry trees are widespread in Midwestern forests. Look for them in hardwood forests growing alongside maples and beeches or along streams.

In late spring, wildcraft flowers, young twigs, and branches to use for tea, tinctures, or infusions. Wildcraft young tips and twigs and the inner bark when the sap runs in the spring to create the best plant bark extract. Collect flowers for a tincture or infusion at the same time. Process the inner bark of the tree in early spring and dry it for later use.

In late summer, harvest the fruit in sunny, dry, and hot weather, which naturally increases the sugars in the cherries. Separate the cherries from the stems and use the fruit immediately, or freeze it for later use.

Wild black cherry fruit is significantly different from that of the cultivated sweet cherry common in the fruit belt of the Midwest; wild cherries are smaller and more tart in flavor. Look for the darkest purple fruits and taste them before wildcrafting the clusters. The variability in the tartness of the fruit (a function of both soil and season) warrants tasting a sample from a particular tree before investing significant time in harvesting. That doesn't mean that even the most sour and bitter cherries would be inedible, however; consider the flavor profile of that batch and have a use for them in mind as you harvest.

Medicinal Uses

Black cherry bark is helpful in relaxing the lungs and respiratory system. Create a cool infusion of the twigs and inner cherry bark to help soothe a spasmodic, barking dry cough. It pairs well with mullein or the soothing inner bark of slippery elm. Use honey to add a soothing sweetness to the tea.

Black cherry flowers and young branch tips have a notable bitter flavor that resembles almond extract when prepared as a tincture. This delicious herbal extract is suited for aromatic and carminative digestive bitters, useful in cases of overindulgence of heavy foods or drinks that leads to excess phlegm in the throat or lungs.

The tincture created from the flowers and twigs can also help open the lungs with environmentally-caused asthma or allergies. It works well with mullein and New England aster for this use.

For a nourishing, antioxidant drink that is high in vitamin C, prepare the fruit as a juice concentrate similar to the commercial concentrate made from cultivated tart cherries, at a fraction of the cost. To make the juice, cover crushed berries (stones and all) in water and simmer them into a rich concentrate. Then strain and bottle the juice or freeze it to use later.

The concentrate is high in antioxidants and has anti-inflammatory properties, making the drink a local superfood. This wild version of cherry juice concentrate can easily replace the commercial concentrate that is popular among athletes as a sports recovery drink.

Future Harvests

Black cherry is widespread in mixed hardwood forests across the Midwest. Use sustainable bark-harvesting practices to prevent the unnecessary destruction of mature trees. Lower hanging berries are abundant, and there is always fruit aplenty for local wildlife on higher branches.

HERBAL PREPARATIONS

Black cherry bark tea
Cool infusion
Drink 1–2 cups as needed.

Black cherry tincture
1 part fresh bark, flowers, and twigs, chopped
2 parts menstruum (95 percent alcohol, 5 percent distilled water)
or
1 part dry bark, flowers, and twigs, chopped
4 parts menstruum (95 percent alcohol, 5 percent distilled water)
Take 25–30 drops as needed.

black walnut

Juglans nigra

PARTS USED hulls

Although the black walnut may be the devil to the home gardener, herbalists value it as an astringent and aromatic bitters that is useful for gastrointestinal imbalances and disorders. Black walnut tincture is helpful to have on hand in a traveler's first aid kit.

How to Identify

Towering walnut trees are abundant in and native to the Midwest. Mature trees can reach 150 feet tall, with trunks 2–3 feet in diameter, but most grow to 80–100 feet.

The gray-black bark is deeply furrowed. Compound leaves comprise up to 23 stemless, oval, serrated leaflets. The walnut flowers in late spring and bears globular fruit—bright green hulls that fully ripen and begin to fall from the trees in late summer. Inside the hull is a hard shell that surrounds the nutmeat, which is usually made up of two halves separated by a thin partition.

Where, When, and How to Wildcraft

Look for walnut trees growing in full sun, often along the edges of the forest. They are also planted in urban landscapes. In late summer and early fall, look for wind-fallen walnuts on sidewalks and streets. Then look up to see the tree.

Wildcraft the green hulls, which are very aromatic, before the squirrels collect them all! As black walnuts ripen, their husks change from solid green to yellowish green. Partially ripened walnuts are also useful, but they may be infested with maggots.

Medicinal Uses

Prepared as a simple tincture or blended with other herbs, black walnut hulls are used as a

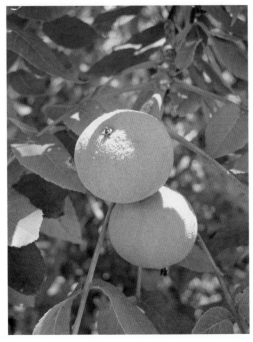

The green hulls of black walnut are aromatic and bitter. Prepared as a simple tincture or as a tincture with other herbs, black walnut can be used as a digestive bitters that has top notes of citrus and vanilla.

digestive bitters that has notes of citrus and vanilla flavors. Consider mixing black walnut hulls with spicebush, tulip poplar, and wild ginger to create an herbal tincture combination that stimulates digestion and soothes an upset stomach from overindulgence. For flu or food poisoning, combine aromatic and

Nocino: A Traditional Herbal Digestif

Not only does black walnut offer delicious nutmeats to include in cooking and baked goods, but the green hull has a fragrant, citrusy aroma that can be infused in alcohol to make nocino, an aromatic and spicy liqueur that is beneficial for digestion. Walnut hulls are the main ingredient in the traditional Italian digestif that also contains clove, orange peel, nutmeg, juniper, and cinnamon.

Traditionally, nocino is made from English walnuts, but here in the Midwest, we can use black walnuts instead. Enjoy your nocino as a sipping liqueur in a dessert course with fragrant cheeses, wild plum cake, and dark chocolate. Experiment with wild spices, including spicebush, tulip poplar, and wild ginger, to create a nocino with real local flavor.

Homemade nocino liqueur

4 quarts of green walnut hulls
1 tablespoon cardamom
1 tablespoon cloves
1 tablespoon ginger
1 tablespoon juniper berries
1 tablespoon orange peel
2 cinnamon sticks
vodka or white wine

1. Quarter the hulls and stuff them, along with the spices, to the brim in several large canning jars.
2. In each jar, cover the mixture completely with vodka (or white wine), and let it sit for 8 weeks.
3. Strain and preserve the liqueur in a glass bottle and let it age, or bottle it into small apothecary dropper bottles to use for traveling.

Take 30–60 drops as needed for acute digestive troubles, or sip as a liqueur.

bitter black walnut hulls with artemisia or lemon balm to help the stomach manage the invading pathogen.

For the first aid kit, a tincture blend of artemisia, black walnut hulls, and lemon balm can help with digestive issues, especially when traveling to countries where water and food quality may affect the stomach.

Future Harvests

Black walnut trees are abundant across the Midwest and are deemed by some as an invasive species. Wildcrafting the hulls for household use will have no impact on the plant's sustainability.

Cautions, Concerns, and Considerations

Walnut hulls are green, but they contain several compounds that create a brownish black stain that dyes anything they touch, including the pavement and your hands. Wear old clothes and latex or vinyl gloves while collecting and processing them.

Black walnut roots, hulls, and leaves secrete juglone, a chemical that inhibits the growth of other nearby plants. For this reason, many garden plants, especially apples, tomatoes, and white birch, should not be planted in proximity of a black walnut. Some

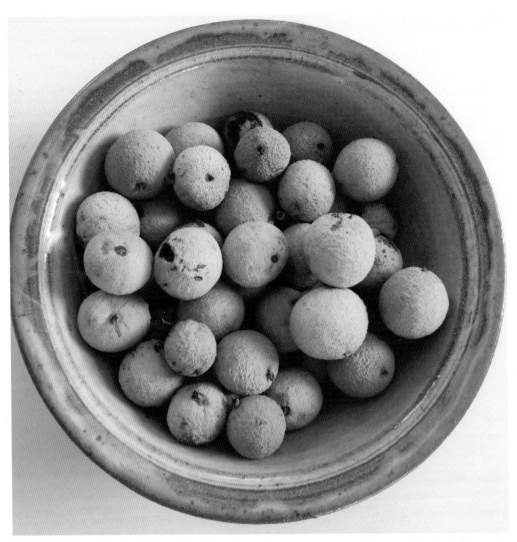

Consider making a black walnut nocino with spicebush, tulip poplar, and wild ginger. This herbal tincture can be used to stimulate digestion and soothe an upset stomach.

literature questions whether the juglone content renders the nut inedible, but there is enough traditional and contemporary use of black walnut to negate this potential concern.

HERBAL PREPARATIONS

Black walnut hull tincture
1 part fresh green hulls, smashed
2 parts menstruum (50 percent alcohol, 50 percent distilled water)
Take 20–30 drops as needed for digestive troubles.

Verbena hastata
PARTS USED flowers, leaves

In today's competitive and stressful work culture, blue vervain is a must-have in the herbal apothecary to smooth away stress resulting from a perfectionist mindset. Blue vervain is not overtly sedative, but it is mildly calming.

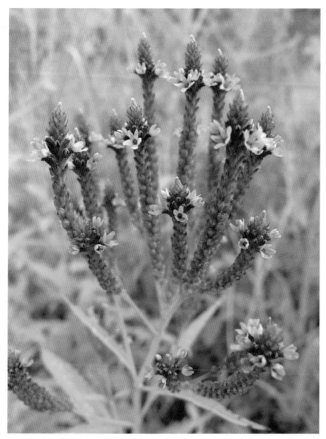

Blue vervain is not overtly sedative, but it is calming. Its bitter flavors can help ease an upset stomach caused by stress and tension, and it also relaxes head and neck tension from computer stress.

How to Identify

Square, hairy stems of perennial blue vervain can grow 2–6 feet tall. Flowers bloom in late summer to early fall on 3- to 6-inch spikes lined with densely clustered, small blue-purple blossoms. Lance-shaped, serrated leaves are 3–5 inches long and are arranged oppositely along the stem. Blue vervain is bitter in flavor and not aromatic.

Where, When, and How to Wildcraft

Blue vervain prefers rich, well-drained soil and commonly grows in streambeds and moist, low-lying fields and wetlands. In high summer, look for its blue flowers in late July and early August, continuing into Labor Day in early September.

Blue vervain is a sun-loving plant. Wildcraft its leaves and blossoms on sunny, warm days in the morning after the dew has dried. Dry the plant stalks in bundles or spread them on screens to dry.

Medicinal Uses

Blue vervain's chief virtue is its use in a relaxant tea that can help ease an upset stomach caused by stress and tension. It also relaxes head and neck tension that can result from computer use.

This is a worthwhile plant to have on hand for tea. Blend it with aromatics such as chamomile and wild rose, which may increase its relaxing effect. Or mix it with lavender, lemon balm, or rose petals.

Future Harvests

Blue vervain is a perennial native plant and is not frequently found in great abundance. Wetland habitat loss is a concern for the sustainability of the plant. When wildcrafting blue vervain, harvest only a few leaves and flowers from each plant.

Cautions, Concerns, and Considerations

Some claim that drinking blue vervain tea can have a nauseating effect. I can see this as a possibility if one drinks successive gallons of the tea or tincture, but because it is extremely bitter in taste, it is not something that would normally be consumed in large quantities.

HERBAL PREPARATIONS

Blue vervain tea
Cold infusion
Drink ¼ cup as needed.

Blue vervain tincture
1 part fresh flowers and leaves, chopped
2 parts menstruum (50 percent alcohol, 50 percent distilled water)
or
1 part dry flowers and leaves, chopped
4 parts menstruum (50 percent alcohol, 50 percent distilled water)
Take 25–30 drops as needed.

boneset

Eupatorium perfoliatum
PARTS USED flowers, leaves

Boneset is a common native wildflower that has held a prominent place in the herbal apothecary for its powerful antiviral properties. Bitter in flavor, boneset is traditionally used in herbal blends and protocols to support the body's defense against viral infections such as influenza, dengue fever, and the West Nile virus.

How to Identify

Boneset is a striking wildflower that grows in stands in rich, well-drained soil. Boneset leaves are thin and lanceolate, up to 8 inches long, arranged oppositely along a hairy, thick central stem that can reach 4 feet tall. White flower clusters bloom in midsummer to early fall and vary in size from 2 to 8 inches across.

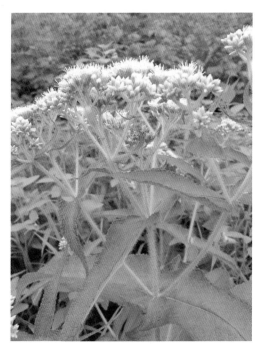

Boneset, bitter in flavor, is traditionally used in herbal blends and protocols to support the body's defense against viral infections like influenza, dengue fever, and the West Nile virus.

The florets are replaced by seed-bearing achenes with small tufts of hair that are dispersed by the wind. One of its chief identifiers is its notably bitter taste.

Where, When, and How to Wildcraft

Look for boneset in fields and hedgerows, growing in the sun and interspersed with other native wildflowers. Harvest leaves and flowers just as the plant begins to bloom in midsummer, as pollinators tend to munch on the plant across the summer. If you miss this harvest window, don't worry. Boneset is resilient enough and is of such value to the apothecary that harvesting even subpar plant material is worth your effort.

Trim the flower clusters and wildcraft leaves from individual plants. If the stand is sizable, wildcraft full stems of the plant and bundle them to dry for later processing into tea.

Medicinal Uses

Boneset is not often used on its own and is commonly blended with black cohosh, elderberry, elderflower, spotted bee balm, wild bergamot, and yarrow in teas and extracts.

Because of its long-standing use and benefits as an herbal remedy for treating viruses and fevers, boneset is a highly valuable plant medicine in the field or apothecary. When used to treat body aches and pains from

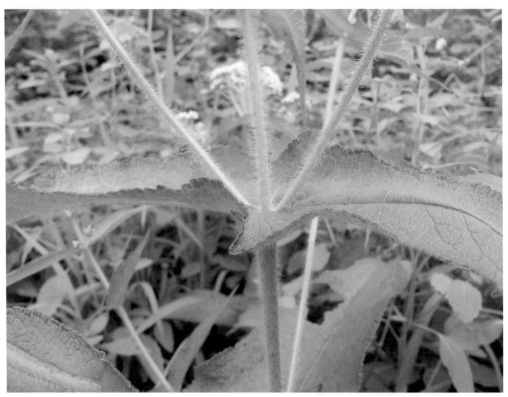

Boneset leaves are united at their bases along the hairy stem, which grows straight through the leaf pair.

fever, boneset is a relaxant and diaphoretic that helps the body produce sweat. Bone-break fever (dengue fever of the South and swamplands, as well as West Nile virus) indicates where boneset can be used as a tea to help allay the aches of the fever without artificially suppressing the body's natural immune functions.

Future Harvests

Boneset is distributed across much of the Midwest in wetlands and swamp areas. Habitat loss is of chief concern to the abundance of boneset. It can be propagated by divisions and replanting in the fall.

Cautions, Concerns, and Considerations

Some claim that boneset tea will have an emetic effect (it will cause vomiting) if consumed in large quantities. This may be possible if a person drinks successive gallons of the tea or tincture. But because boneset is markedly bitter, it is not something normally consumed in large quantities. Instead, it is usually blended as part of a more complex herbal protocol to support the body's immune response during viral illness.

HERBAL PREPARATIONS

Boneset tea
Infusion
Drink ¼ cup.

Boneset tincture
1 part fresh flowers and leaves, chopped
2 parts menstruum (50 percent alcohol,
   50 percent distilled water)
or
1 part dry flowers and leaves, chopped
4 parts menstruum (50 percent alcohol,
   50 percent distilled water)
*Take 10–15 drops, 3 to 5 times during acute
illness.*

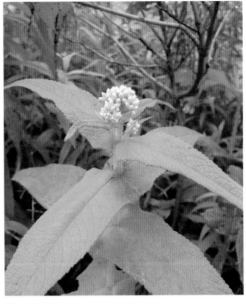

Boneset blossoms are starting to open.

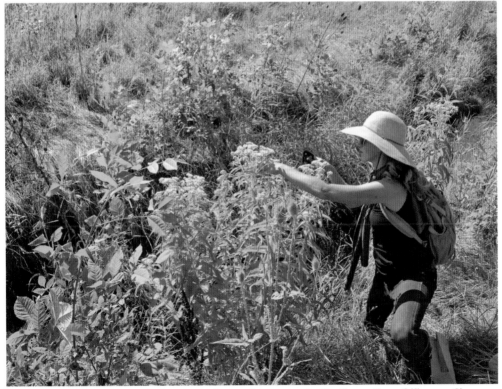

Look for boneset in fields and hedgerows in the sun, interspersed with other native wildflowers. Choose to wildcraft boneset just as it begins to bloom in midsummer.

borage

Borago officinalis
PARTS USED flowers, leaves

Borage is useful in the apothecary for making a cooling and refreshing summer tea and easing melancholy and sadness.

How to Identify

Borage is a native Mediterranean garden herb that has naturalized in the Midwest. It commonly reseeds and often grows outside cultivated gardens. In fact, borage reproduces prolifically and is considered an invasive plant.

This annual prefers sun and tolerates poor soil. The whole plant, which grows 2–3 feet tall, is covered in stiff, prickly hairs. Hairy

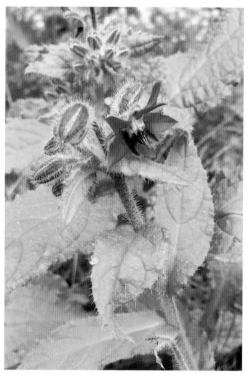

As an herbal medicine, borage is traditionally used to dispel melancholy, sadness, and grief.

oblong leaves are arranged alternately along the succulent stems. Fresh leaves taste similar to cucumber but lose their flavor when dried.

Borage begins flowering in early summer and blooms in successions throughout the summer. Blossoms are blue or purple, but they can also be white and light pink. Each star-shaped flower has five triangular and pointed petals. Honey bees are drawn to its nectar. The plant dies back after blooming.

Where, When, and How to Wildcraft

Look for borage growing in untended areas as well as in cultivated gardens. Wildcraft leaves and blossoms in the late spring and early summer when the plant is in full bloom. Use borage fresh or wildcraft the entire plant and hang it to dry for later use.

Medicinal Uses

Borage is traditionally used as a plant medicine to dispel melancholy, sadness, and grief. A chilled infusion of fresh borage is useful in this way, as is a tincture of borage with other heart-healing herbs such as hawthorn, lemon balm, and rose. Flower essences of borage can also be prepared for this use.

Combine borage with lemon balm and rose petals to make a lovely and cooling herbal tea. Serve chilled with lemon and honey.

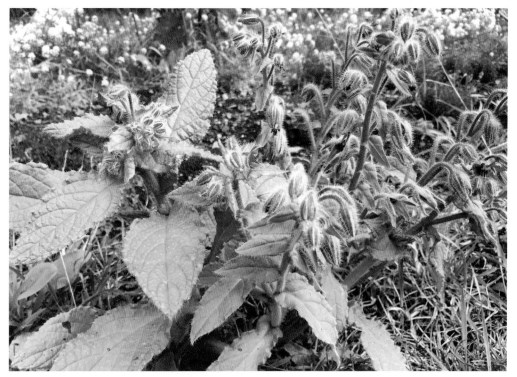

Use fresh borage leaves and flowers to make a delightful cucumber-flavored cold infusion for a calming and refreshing herbal tea on a hot summer day.

Future Harvests

Borage aggressively reproduces and spreads rapidly. Wildcrafting leaves and flowers will do little to affect the plant's distribution.

Cautions, Concerns, and Considerations

Like coltsfoot and comfrey, borage contains alkaloids which research has found to cause liver damage when consumed in high concentrations. Use this herb only with supervision by a trained practitioner.

HERBAL PREPARATIONS

Borage tea
Cold infusion
1 part fresh flowers and leaves, chopped
Drink 1 cup.

Borage tincture
1 part fresh flowers and leaves, chopped
2 parts menstruum (50 percent alcohol,
   50 percent distilled water)
Take 8–10 drops as needed.

burdock

Arctium species

PARTS USED roots

Although burdock is cursed by many as an invasive weed, it is a valuable and versatile wild food and medicine that grows in abundance around us. Burdock root is used for its ability to help the body regulate the metabolism.

How to Identify

Burdock is a drought-tolerant, hardy biennial plant that thrives in many conditions, including poor and rocky soils. It grows along the disturbed edges of fields and waste sites and is prolific in spreading seeds.

First-year burdock is identifiable by its large, triangular, fuzzy basal leaves that resemble rhubarb leaves. In the second year, burdock takes a bushier form and sends up a sturdy branched stalk, 2–5 feet tall. The prickly heads, or burs, that form on the stalk are composite flowers that bloom in late spring to midsummer.

Where, When, and How to Wildcraft

Burdock grows virtually everywhere across the Midwest. It is known for its sturdy and nutritious taproot that affixes the plant solidly to the ground. Select a harvest area that has soft, rich, and well-drained soil, and wildcraft the root in the spring or fall.

The first-year root is easiest to wildcraft, but a second-year root is also edible (although potentially woody). Bring a spade and be prepared for some serious digging, especially with second-year plants, because the taproot can be quite long and deep. Dig in a wide circumference to avoid shearing off the taproot.

In the kitchen, scrub the root clean. Wild burdock roots are much more gnarled than roots of its cultivated counterpart, gobō, or

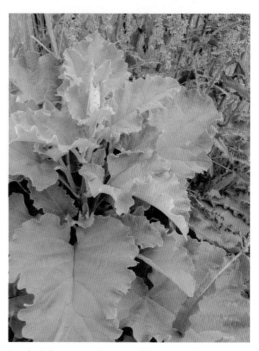

Burdock leaves are large and fuzzy, with wavy margins.

greater burdock (*Arctium lappa*), and small pockets can retain a significant amount of soil. To prepare the clean root for tea, chop it into small pieces, dry it completely in a dehydrator, and store in an airtight container. Fresh or dry roots can also be prepared as a tincture.

Medicinal Uses

Burdock root is useful for people afflicted by modern-day stress and for those who have

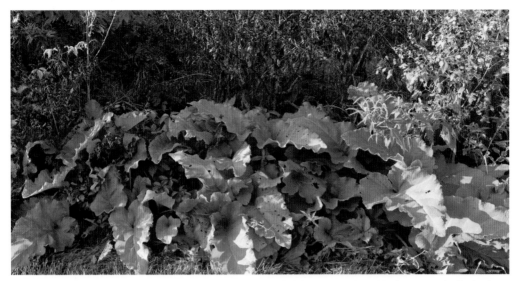

Burdock root is most known and used as a metabolic tonic. Also a nourishing food, it can help the body restore tone to the digestive system.

depressed digestive systems. It offers support for the liver and restores stagnant digestion. Not only is burdock a nourishing food, but it can boost the digestive system by helping the body absorb and eliminate foods.

Burdock root is especially helpful when used as part of a protocol for those whose stagnant digestion is expressed in the body as eczema, dry skin, or regular acne break-outs. (It's worthwhile to research potential food allergies in this case as well and work on stimulating digestion.) In these cases, a tincture of burdock root is most effective as part of a daily herbal digestive protocol.

Burdock works well as a decoction with warming, carminative herbs to support digestion, including cinnamon, clove, and other metabolic and lymphatic tonics such as ceanothus, dandelion root, and yellow dock. For a warming and stimulating aromatic chai tea, toast dehydrated burdock roots in an iron skillet and combine them with roasted chaga, chicory root, dandelion root, hickory nuts, and spicebush.

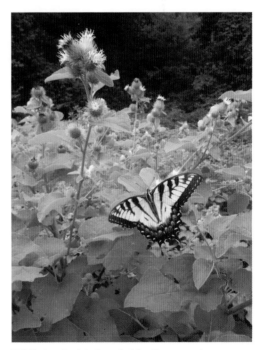

While burdock is found virtually everywhere across the Midwest, take care in selecting a harvest area with softer, rich, well-drained soil. Especially in urban and suburban areas, be sure it is free of herbicidal applications, lead, or environmental pollutants.

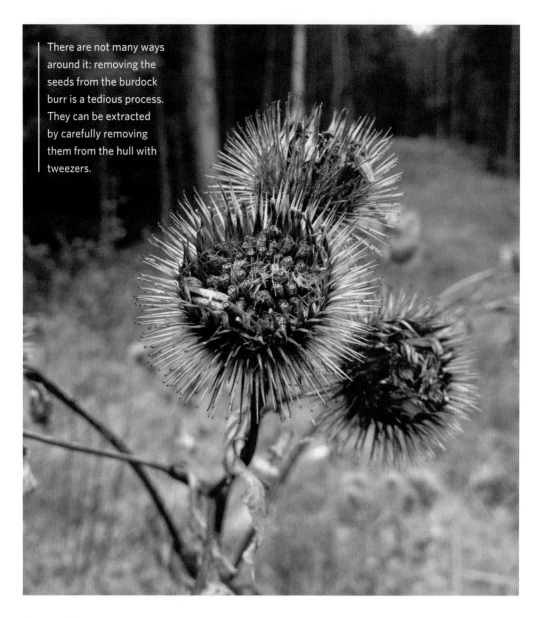

There are not many ways around it: removing the seeds from the burdock burr is a tedious process. They can be extracted by carefully removing them from the hull with tweezers.

Future Harvests

Burdock is considered a noxious weed by many, but perhaps if we relearn its virtues, focus will shift to the value the plant provides. Currently, however, burdock is subject to aggressive plant management strategies by gardeners, farmers, and park groundskeepers. A partnership opportunity is waiting to grow between the medicine-makers and land stewards who want to manage the growth and use of this plant sustainably, but currently there is little concern about overharvesting.

Cautions, Concerns, and Considerations

Because burdock grows abundantly in urban and suburban areas and is sometimes

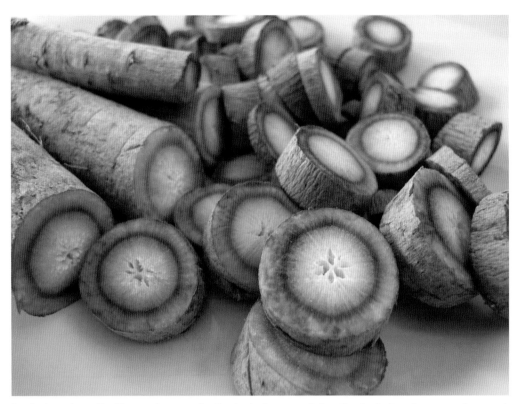

Burdock works well with warming, carminative herbs to support digestion including cinnamon, clove, and other metabolic and lymphatic tonics like ceanothus, dandelion root, and yellow dock.

considered a weed, be sure the harvesting area is free of herbicidal applications, lead contamination, or environmental pollutants. To identify a clean spot for harvesting, contact a local organic farmer; chances are burdock is growing on his or her land, and the farmer will be more than happy to allow you to do some digging (just remember to backfill the holes).

HERBAL PREPARATIONS

Burdock root tea
Decoction
Drink 1 cup per day.

Burdock root tincture
1 part fresh root, chopped
2 parts menstruum (50 percent alcohol, 50 percent distilled water)
or
1 part dry root, chopped
4 parts menstruum (50 percent alcohol, 50 percent distilled water)
Take 25 drops per day.

Asclepias tuberosa
pleurisy root
PARTS USED roots

Butterfly weed is a relaxant medicinal plant that's useful in easing wet, damp, and constricted lung ailments.

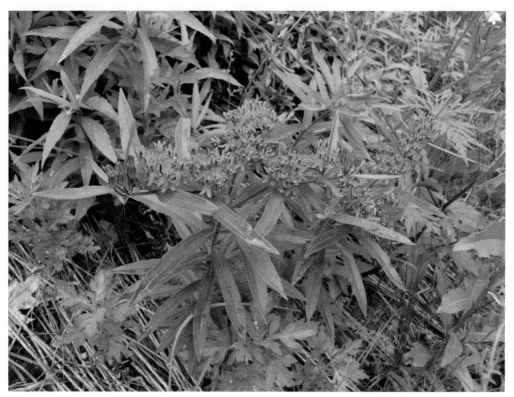

Butterfly weed tolerates poor soil and thrives in damp conditions. Wildcraft the roots in the early spring or fall, after the plant is done blooming.

How to Identify

Butterfly weed is a perennial plant with 12- to 36-inch-tall, upright, hairy stems. Deep green, lance-shaped leaves are arranged alternately. Flat-topped, 2- to 5-inch clusters (umbels) of tiny flowers are showy in midsummer, in vibrant orange to orange-red colors.

Where, When, and How to Wildcraft

Find butterfly weed growing in full sun in damp fields with poor soils. Wildcraft the roots in the early spring or fall, after the plant is done blooming. The roots should be cleaned and used fresh or dried for tincture or tea.

Medicinal Uses

Butterfly weed root is a slightly bitter-tasting lymphatic medicine that can help relax damp and constrictive lung ailments. It can stimulate movement of damp congestion in the lungs and supports productive elimination of stuck, excess mucus.

When used in a cold infusion or tincture, butterfly weed can ease a damp, persistent cough and blends well with other herbs such as boneset, goldenrod, mullein, slippery elm, and yarrow, depending on the condition treated. To offset the bitterness of butterfly weed root tea, sweeten it with honey, which is a helpful antimicrobial that offers additional soothing for inflamed tissues.

Future Harvests

Butterfly weed is a native plant loved by honey bees, hummingbirds, butterflies, and other pollinators. Because of habitat loss, keep sustainability in mind as you remove entire plants to collect the roots. Choose to help propagate the plant in other wild areas and in cultivated gardens or permaculture plantings.

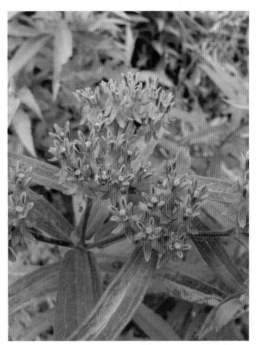

Butterfly weed is a slightly bitter lymphatic that can help relax damp and constrictive lung ailments. The orange flowers are a nectar source for many butterflies, and its leaves are a food source for monarch butterfly larvae.

HERBAL PREPARATIONS

Butterfly weed tea
Cold infusion
Drink ¼ cup as needed.

Butterfly weed tincture
1 part fresh roots, chopped
2 parts menstruum (50 percent alcohol,
   50 percent distilled water)
or
1 part dry roots, chopped
4 parts menstruum (50 percent alcohol,
   50 percent distilled water)
Take 25 drops, 3 to 5 times per day.

calamus

Acorus calamus
bitter-root, sweet-flag
PARTS USED leaves, rhizomes

The spicy, bitter, and fragrant notes of calamus can help clear a busy mind and settle an upset stomach. This amazing herb can help restore balance to an imbalanced system.

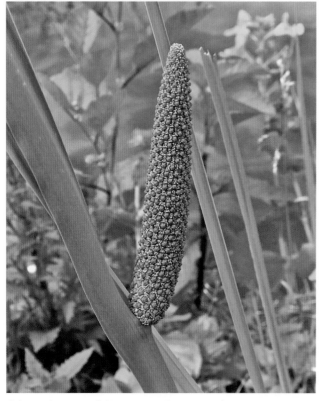

Calamus leaves and rhizomes can be prepared as a tea, tincture, massage oil, or essential oil, or simply chewed. To calm a busy and unsettled mind, simply chew on the dried rhizome.

How to Identify

This grasslike perennial grows similarly to iris, with long, sword-shaped leaves up to 5 feet in length, with noticeable midribs and veins. Calamus produces a triangular scape (a long, leafless stem) at the base of the outer leaves, which sends up a 2- to 4-inch spadix, or spike, in early summer that is covered in tiny yellow and brown flowers.

Calamus produces rhizomes, white and brown underground stems that spread below the soil. The entire plant smells of spicy citrus, and the leaves are notably scented when crushed.

Where, When, and How to Wildcraft

Look for calamus growing in damp soils along muddy stream banks and wetlands throughout the Midwest. Wildcraft young leaves in spring for tea or chewing. Wildcraft the rhizomes in the early spring or late fall after the plant has flowered.

Medicinal Uses

You can prepare calamus in many ways—as a tea, tincture, massage oil, or essential oil. To calm a busy and unsettled mind, chew on the dried rhizome. Notice the bitter shudder that helps call attention to the breath and demands a sense of presence. Its bitter aromatics clear the senses to help a cloudy mind become free of clutter.

For the stomach, chewing calamus leaves or rhizome or using a calamus tincture can help stimulate stagnant digestion. Its aromatic nature acts as a carminative on the digestive system and can quell stomach bloating and dispel gas.

As a bitters, calamus can be prepared as a simple tincture that helps stimulate digestion, or blend it with other herbs such as burdock, ceanothus, lemon balm, spicebush, wild bergamot, and yellow dock to help stimulate and support the body's metabolism and lymphatic systems.

Future Harvests

Select rhizomes from established stands, and help grow more plants by planting rhizome cuttings. Seeds can also be planted in late fall. Consider adding calamus to rain gardens and other permaculture designs.

Cautions, Concerns, and Considerations

Although large doses of calamus may overstimulate the system and cause vomiting, the history and ethnobotanical use of calamus suggests it is safe for herbal and culinary uses. Although the US Food and Drug Administration has listed calamus as a carcinogen in mice and states that it should not be consumed internally, these conclusions are based on chemical extractions of active ingredients that are injected in large doses into laboratory animals.

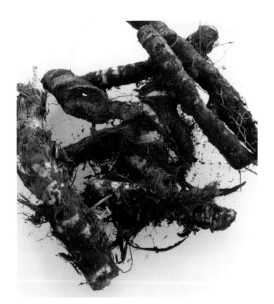

For the stomach, chewing the bitter calamus root or using the tincture can help stimulate stagnant digestion. Calamus can be used fresh or dry.

HERBAL PREPARATIONS

Calamus tea
Infusion
Drink ¼ cup as needed.

Calamus tincture
1 part fresh leaves and rhizomes, chopped
2 parts menstruum (50 percent alcohol,
   50 percent distilled water)
or
1 part dry leaves and rhizomes, chopped
4 parts menstruum (50 percent alcohol,
   50 percent distilled water)
Take 8–10 drops as needed.

Calamus-infused oil
1 part fresh leaves and rhizomes, chopped
2 parts oil
or
1 part dry leaves and rhizomes, chopped
4 parts oil
Use for massage.

catnip

Nepeta cataria
catmint
PARTS USED flowers, leaves

A valuable herbal remedy, catnip can be used to make digestive bitters. This nervine (nerve-calming) and relaxant herb is helpful for both smooth tissues and skeletal muscles and tissues. Its aromatic properties make it an effective bug repellant.

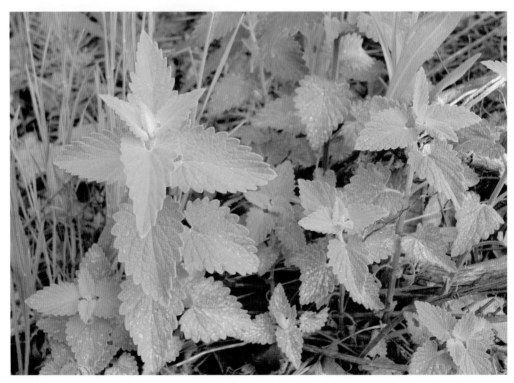

Catnip is a clumping, dusty green, mint family plant. It stands about 2 to 3 feet tall with soft and downy heart-shaped leaves oppositely arranged on its square stems.

How to Identify

Catnip is a clumping, dusty green, and hairy plant in the mint family. It stands 2–3 feet tall with soft and downy heart-shaped leaves oppositely arranged on square stems. The plant is small and tender through mid-summer, when it sends up a dense spike of blossoms that range in color from white to pinkish and even a deep purple (especially the garden cultivars).

Where, When, and How to Wildcraft

Catnip is a rough-and-tumble plant—it doesn't mind scrubby, nutrient-depleted soil,

Keep the Bugs Away with Botanicals

Summertime means camping trips, picnics, and time spent at the lakeshore surrounded by family and friends. Unwelcome visitors often attend the festivities, too, including pesky mosquitos, ticks, and spiders, all unavoidable in our forests and backyards.

Although you'll find many commercially made chemical-free bug sprays to help deter bugs and soothe bothersome bug bites, they can be pricey. Consider making your own blends of herbal bug repellants from tinctures you've created. Plant-based alternatives help keep the bugs away and keep the itching at bay, and they're easy to make at home by mixing a few plant tinctures with distilled water. Spritz the spray on clothing and skin to deter bugs and use it topically to soothe bites.

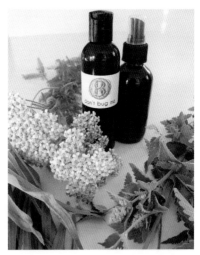

The plant extracts of catnip work effectively in an herbal bug spray blend with chickweed, plantain, and yarrow.

Herbal bug spray

1 part catnip tincture
1 part chickweed tincture
1 part plantain tincture
1 part yarrow tincture

1. Combine the tinctures.
2. Add 1 part tincture mix to 1 part distilled water and pour it into a spray bottle.
3. Add 15 drops of essential oils of lavender or lemongrass, as preferred, per 4 ounces of bottled spray.

and it often grows in sunny vacant lots in urban areas. You'll also find catnip growing along the edges of grassy fields and hedgerows near parks, gardens, and farms.

To preserve the plant's aromatic qualities, harvest the plants when they are fully dry. Wildcraft full stalks in early summer before they bloom, and then bundle and hang the stalks to dry for tea. Harvest the blossoms in midsummer to use fresh or dry them for later use. Store dry flowers and leaves in airtight containers.

Medicinal Uses

Catnip is the most relaxant of the mint plants. It is oily and aromatic like other mints but is notably skunky in aroma and bitter in taste.

Its relaxant property helps soothe an upset stomach (particularly with vomiting—take small sips of tea), dispel gas, and soothe stomach constriction and tension. As a stomach bitters, catnip can be prepared alone in tea or blended with wildcrafted burdock root, tulip poplar, and wild ginger.

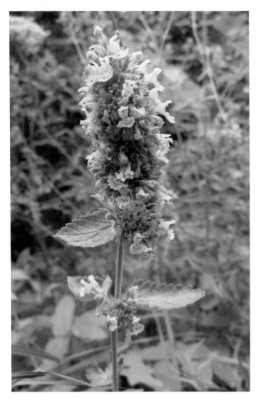

The relaxant property of catnip can help soothe an upset stomach, dispel gas, and relieve stomach constriction and tension.

Catnip tea is mild enough for wee ones with stomach upsets or who have trouble sleeping. To minimize the bitter flavors, make catnip tea with cool water and serve it over ice with lemon. Add a sprig of lavender and a dollop of raw honey.

When sipped as a warm tea, catnip relaxes the body and supports a productive fever over the course of an illness such as a cold or influenza. It blends well with boneset, elderflower, peppermint, spotted bee balm, wild bergamot, and yarrow.

Extract catnip's leaves and flowers into an oil for massage to soothe skeletal muscle pain resulting from muscle spasms or cramps, or use it for a neck massage oil. The tea can also be added to a soothing bath with Epsom salts for a post-exercise muscle soak; this works nicely with wildcrafted meadowsweet flowers mixed in.

Future Harvests

Catnip is a common wild plant and considered a weed by many. The perennial catnip you identify this season will be there next season provided you haven't harvested the entire plant. Harvest the aerial parts of the plant in moderation. To grow a stand of catnip, propagate plants from cuttings from the parent plant.

HERBAL PREPARATIONS

Catnip tea
Infusion
Drink ¼ cup as needed.

Catnip tincture
1 part fresh flowers and leaves, chopped
2 parts menstruum (50 percent alcohol,
   50 percent distilled water)
or
1 part dry flowers and leaves, chopped
4 parts menstruum (50 percent alcohol,
   50 percent distilled water)
Take 15 drops as needed.

Catnip-infused oil
1 part fresh flowers and leaves, chopped
2 parts oil
or
1 part dry flowers and leaves, chopped
4 parts oil
Use for massage.

---

ceanothus

Ceanothus americanus
New Jersey tea, red root
PARTS USED inner bark, roots

The blood-red extract of ceanothus bark and roots acts on the stomach as an astringent digestive aid and supports metabolic processes. It is an excellent remedy to include in a traveler's first aid kit.

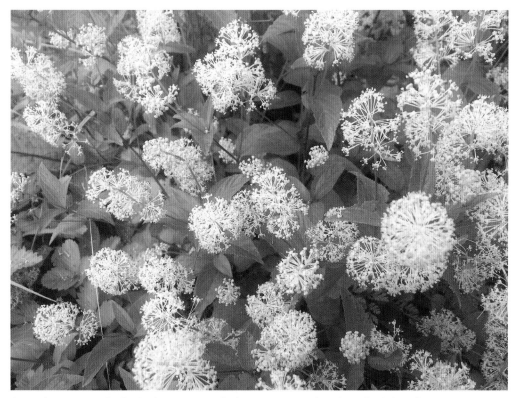

Ceanothus is a woody shrub whose roots make for an important lymphatic herbal medicine.

How to Identify

Ceanothus is a woody shrub that grows 2–3 feet tall. Pale to dark-green foliage grows along the stem in both alternate and opposite arrangements. Leaves are about 3 inches long and 2 inches wide, ovate, finely serrated, and deeply veined, with short petioles. In midsummer, stalks bear showy white terminal clusters of flowers. The plant has a slight floral fragrance.

Where, When, and How to Wildcraft

Ceanothus prefers fertile, well-drained soil but tolerates poor and rocky soil. It often grows along rock outcrops, in fields, and in open prairies.

Wildcraft the roots in early spring or late fall when the plant is dormant. Use a pickax to dig out small sections of roots for tincture. The plant's dark red inner bark can also be wildcrafted in early spring, but taste it for astringency and experiment for the best results.

Medicinal Uses

The blood-red root and bark extract of ceanothus is a lymphatic and astringent herb. This helpful digestive aid supports the metabolic and lymphatic processes to clear excess loads on the system caused by heavy foods, environmental allergens, illness, and stress.

Ceanothus works by engaging the lymphatic system to help with the removal of body wastes. This is especially important in the late stages of an illness or infection or with a chronic condition, when the immune and lymphatic systems need a boost to clear out the waste by-products of the illness.

Ceanothus also works well in combination with echinacea to turn the tides of systemic infections. Used aggressively with mastitis, for example, these two herbs (with a small amount of poke root tincture) can help unplug stagnant milk ducts in the breast almost immediately and relieves pressure and discomfort for the nursing mother.

Ceanothus can stimulate digestion in combination with calming bitters such as lemon balm or warming bitters such as cinnamon or orange peel. I like to use ceanothus tincture after eating a big bowl of ice cream. A few drops of tincture help my stomach process and clear the damp, dairy belly-ache that comes from my overindulgence.

As an astringent, ceanothus can be used topically as a wash to dry up wet and weepy rashes caused by poison ivy and other toxic plants. Here again, it combines well with echinacea.

Future Harvests

Ceanothus is a perennial shrub, so wildcrafting the roots can disturb the plant. Harvest roots in moderation to avoid affecting the plant population. Plants can be propagated by cuttings and added to a permaculture or medicinal garden.

HERBAL PREPARATIONS

Ceanothus tea
Decoction
Drink ¼ cup, or use externally as an astringent wound wash.

Ceanothus tincture
1 part fresh roots and inner bark, chopped
2 parts menstruum (95 percent alcohol,
    5 percent distilled water)
or
1 part dry roots and inner bark, chopped
4 parts menstruum (95 percent alcohol,
    5 percent distilled water)
Take 15 drops as needed.

---

chaga

Inonotus obliquus
PARTS USED fruiting body

Chaga is an important functional medicine for the apothecary to help modulate and boost the immune system. It also tastes like chocolate.

How to Identify

Chaga is a tough, woody parasitic fungus that grows out of wounds in birch trees. With a seasoned eye, you will begin to recognize chaga fruiting bodies across the seasons. What looks like a burl on the birch is actually the sclerotia, a gnarled expression of the fruit of the fungus. Its dark black, craggy exterior looks a bit like charcoal, but inside, the fungus is reddish brown.

Where, When, and How to Wildcraft

Chaga grows in forests across the Northern Hemisphere; in the Midwest, look for chaga in areas where birch trees are plentiful. Harvest it in the late fall and winter, after birch trees have gone dormant for winter and the chaga is at its nutritional peak. You can harvest it throughout the winter until the tree sap starts running in early spring. Although chaga can be harvested at any time of year, spring- and summer-harvested chaga contains more water and fewer nutrients.

Bring along a mallet or small hammer, hand ax, or hacksaw to remove the chaga from the tree. It is very sturdy material! Remove only the external part of the fungus so the inner fruiting body can continue to digest the decaying birch tree and regrow a new fruiting body.

Chaga takes three to five years to reach a harvestable size. Once harvested, chaga can take up to a decade to regrow to a harvestable size. Practice mindful harvesting techniques and do not remove the entire fruiting body from the tree.

A Warming Herbal Masala Chai

Chai is one of my favorite warming drinks. This wonderful beverage can help move circulation to fingers and toes when the weather turns colder.

My base recipe for chai is a masala blend made up of kitchen spices. Adding chaga to the masala chai blend provides a deep chocolate flavor along with the immune-boosting benefits that come from the mushroom. For an exceptional local chai, replace the kitchen herbs with acorn hulls, beechnuts, chicory roots, sassafras roots, spicebush, wild burdock roots, and wild ginger.

Chaga masala chai

1 tablespoon ground cinnamon
1 tablespoon whole cloves
1 tablespoon whole coriander
½ tablespoon ground cumin
¼ tablespoon whole black pepper
¼ tablespoon whole cardamom
¼ tablespoon whole ginger
dash of ground nutmeg
2 tablespoons ground chaga
black tea
maple syrup or honey

1. Dry toast the masala spices (cinnamon through ginger) in an iron skillet on the stove. After the blend cools, add a dash of nutmeg, and then grind the spice mixture in a grinder.
2. Add the masala spice blend and chaga powder to a pot and cover with 2 quarts of boiling water. Simmer for 20 minutes.
3. Remove from the heat. Add equal parts masala-chaga blend and black tea to a cup and steep to the desired strength. I like to use lapsang souchong. Sweeten the chai with maple syrup or local honey. Add a dollop of local cream if you like. Sip and enjoy.

Makes 2 quarts

In the kitchen, chaga is nearly impossible to process without using heavy tools, such as a hammer and a wood rasp, to break it up and grind it down to a fine powder for infusions. You might want to wear protective eyewear as you work, lest chunks of flying chaga land in your eye.

To process large chaga, break it into chunks and use a sizable, durable mortar and pestle to break it into smaller pieces. Don't put entire chaga pieces in your blender or spice grinder, because the tough pieces will likely burn out the motor and ruin the blades. Use a wood rasp to grate the chaga to a fine powder. Some suggest that the black exterior of the mushroom should be removed, but I use the whole thing.

Medicinal Uses
Chaga helps boost the foundational immune system and provides nutrition to cells and tissues. The polysaccharides of the

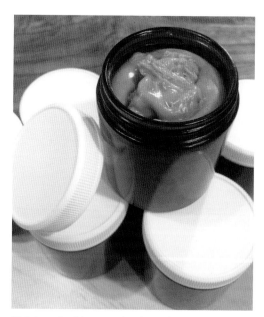

Rich in antioxidants and polysaccharides, chaga can be included in a skin-restoring cream.

mushroom are best extracted by simmering chaga in water for about 45 minutes to make a decoction that you can drink as tea.

Chaga has a deliciously rich aroma and tastes like dark chocolate. As a functional food, ground or powdered chaga can be added directly to a tomato-based sauce, chili, or chocolate-and-peanut butter–based dessert or smoothie (or add it to a chocolate flourless cake or black bean brownie).

Chaga is delicious when added to boiled stovetop coffee or chai, providing deep chocolate notes to the brew. It also makes a fine hot chocolate when mixed with cacao. Local beer brewers are starting to add chaga to brews of porters and stouts to add chocolate flavor. For brewing, it pairs well with other flavoring agents such as hops without adding an overly flavored aspect to the brew.

Future Harvests

Because chaga is becoming popular and has been qualified as a locavore superfood, sustainable and careful harvesting of the fungus is important. Practice mindful harvesting techniques and do not remove the entire fruiting body from the tree to ensure that chaga will continue to grow and mature for future harvests. It can take up to a decade for chaga to regrow to a harvestable size.

HERBAL PREPARATIONS

Chaga tea
Decoction
Drink ¼ cup as needed.

chickweed

Stellaria media

PARTS USED flowers, leaves, stems

Chickweed is a helpful plant for the herbal apothecary. What some call a weed is abundant, easy to wildcraft, and effective as a tissue-healer for abrasions and wounds.

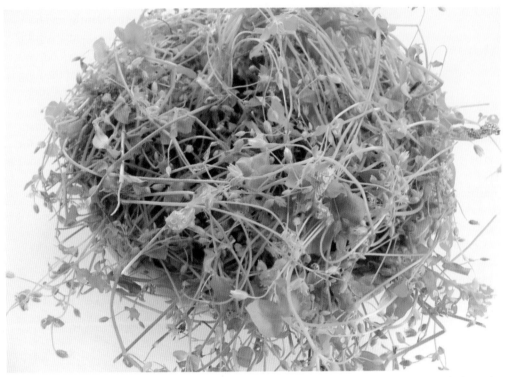

Chickweed is an excellent tissue healer for skin abrasions and wounds. All aerial parts of the chickweed are used.

How to Identify

Chickweed is a low-growing, mat-forming spring annual that thrives in nutrient-rich, well-drained soil. Its small leaves are arranged oppositely on slender stems. Late-spring–blooming white flowers have five deeply notched petals.

Hold a cutting of chickweed up to the light, and you will notice its chief (and fun) identifier: a single line of hairs that runs along the side of the stem. To see the fine hairs better, use a magnifying glass or loupe.

Where, When, and How to Wildcraft

Chickweed creeps along the rich soils of well-composted fields of farms and gardens. It thrives in cool, moist weather and is most vibrant in the height of spring (May), when

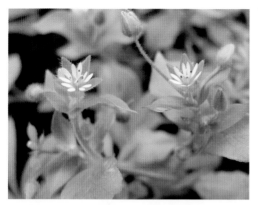

Chickweed is a low-growing, creeping green that can be found in rich soil in mid- to late spring. The tiny stamens of chickweed flowers have reddish violet anthers.

its stems, leaves, and flowers are ready for harvest. In mid-June, it begins to die back, but it returns with a new leaf crop in late fall with the arrival of rains and cooler weather; that growth is not usually as vibrant as the spring crop, however.

Harvest chickweed with kitchen shears in the field—the stems, leaves, and flowers are all edible. Harvest only clean plant material, because chickweed can easily collect dust and debris or mud as it grows along the ground, and it can be difficult to clean completely in the kitchen.

Medicinal Uses

Chickweed is used by herbalists in preparations to heal skin abrasions and wounds. Prepare it as a tincture to take internally for external healing or infuse it in oil to create a base for salve.

When chickweed is being infused in oil, it smells notably swampy. As long as you follow the basic directions for preparing the oil, you need not be concerned. The odor isn't an indicator of a rancid oil; it's just how the chickweed smells. This smell dissipates when the oil is blended into a beeswax salve.

Although an oil-based preparation should never be used in a wet and weepy wound or skin condition, you can use a chickweed preparation as a skin abrasion dries and heals, to help speed up the process. It also works well with other tissue-healing herbs such as calendula, comfrey, plantain, rose, and St. John's wort.

Future Harvests

Chickweed self-sows abundantly, and harvesting its leaves and flowers won't significantly harm its ability to reproduce. In fact, if you plant chickweed in your garden, it readily spreads and can take over very quickly.

HERBAL PREPARATIONS

Chickweed tea
Infusion
Drink ¼ cup, or use externally for topical skin wash.

Chickweed tincture
1 part fresh leaves, chopped
2 parts menstruum (50 percent alcohol, 50 percent distilled water)
or
1 part dry leaves, chopped
4 parts menstruum (50 percent alcohol, 50 percent distilled water)
Take 15 drops per day.

Chickweed-infused oil
1 part fresh leaves, chopped
2 parts oil
or
1 part dry leaves, chopped
4 parts oil
Use for massage.

cleavers

Galium aparine
bedstraw
PARTS USED flowers, leaves, stems

Cleavers is a nourishing spring-cleaning food and herbal remedy for the body.
Not only is it high in vitamin C and chlorophyll, but it's an excellent springtime
lymphatic herb that can help clear swollen glands and lymph nodes.

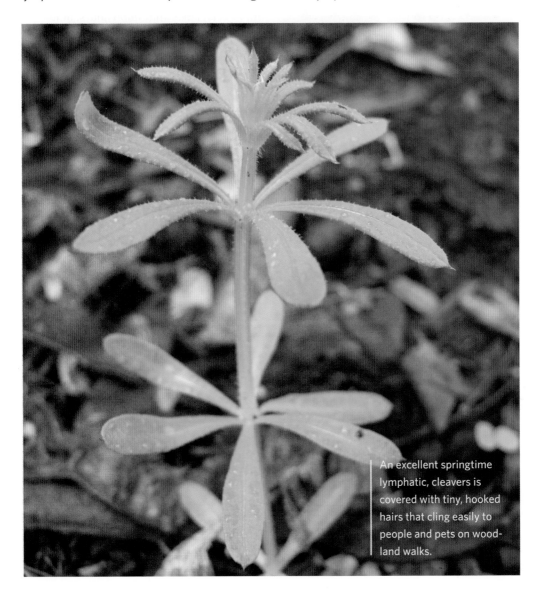

An excellent springtime lymphatic, cleavers is covered with tiny, hooked hairs that cling easily to people and pets on woodland walks.

How to Identify

Cleavers is a sprawling annual that creeps along the ground and over other plants. Its leggy, square stems can reach 3 feet long or more. Six to eight small leaves grow in each whorl on the stem and are narrowly linear in shape. In midspring, cleavers produces petite four-petaled white to greenish flowers. Fuzzy, lobed seed-bearing fruit the size of a small pea are also covered with sticky hairs that cling to animal fur to aid in seed dispersal.

Where, When, and How to Wildcraft

In the early spring, the leaf whorls of cleavers emerge and begin to sprawl across the ground and over low foliage. Look for them in the shady edges of wooded areas, where they grow in rich, damp soil.

Wildcraft the tender whorls as they emerge from early spring until they start to go to seed and die back in late spring. Harvest them by hand or use kitchen shears; or you can easily pull the plant completely out of the ground. Cleavers roots aren't firmly attached to the soil and usually dislodge easily. The whole plant can be used at that point. Try to harvest as little soil as possible, because the sticky hairs make cleavers difficult to clean.

Medicinal Uses

Cleavers is an excellent springtime lymphatic herb. For a nourishing tonic, add cleavers to a springtime tea infusion with nettle, oatstraw, and red clover. Cleavers has a dry and fresh green flavor. Because it is very dry and rough in texture, especially as the plant matures, it is unsuitable for use as salad greens.

Cleavers is full of chlorophyll and vitamin C and makes a good addition to a green smoothie recipe, or juice it as you would wheatgrass. Freeze shots of cleavers juice in ice cube trays for later use in blended drinks. An infusion or tea of cleavers is diuretic, so take this into consideration when using it.

Use fresh cleavers as a topical compress for swollen glands and lymph nodes, or in cases of mastitis. Freeze cleavers to use across the season for lymphatic compresses.

Future Harvests

Cleavers grows abundantly in the springtime and is vigorous in its ability to self-seed. Wildcrafting the plant even in abundance won't significantly impact its sustainability.

HERBAL PREPARATIONS

Cleavers tea
Decoction
Drink 1 cup per day, or use externally as a compress.

Cleavers tincture
1 part fresh leaves, chopped
2 parts menstruum (50 percent alcohol, 50 percent distilled water)
or
1 part dry leaves, chopped
4 parts menstruum (50 percent alcohol, 50 percent distilled water)
Take 25 drops per day.

Tussilago farfara

PARTS USED flowers, leaves, roots, stalks

Coltsfoot is an early spring herb that works wonders to relieve a stubborn spring chest cold and cough. Use fresh or dry plant material in the kitchen to make a strong tea or relaxant syrup for a cough and deep chest cold.

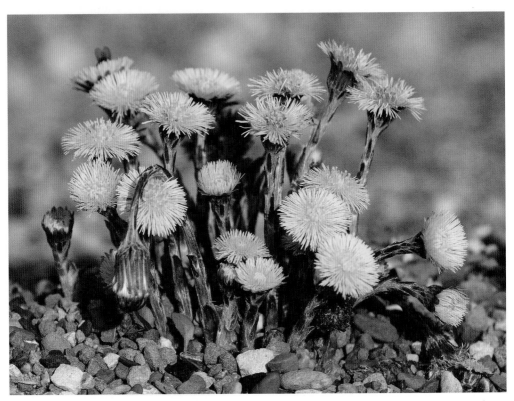

The flowers of coltsfoot emerge before the leaves. This differs from the dandelion, which blooms at the same time as a rosette of leaves at its base.

How to Identify

Coltsfoot is a succulent perennial that sends up stalks and flowers in early spring. Each foot-long stalk has reddish scales and is topped by a single yellow, flat flower that resembles a dandelion bloom. Dark green, heart-shaped leaves emerge in late spring after the plant flowers.

Where, When, and How to Wildcraft

In the early spring, look carefully beneath last season's leaf litter in the damp soils of the woods and you'll find coltsfoot's bright yellow flowers. You can also find it growing on steep road cuts, where the soil has been exposed. Here, coltsfoot helps hold the soil in place to prevent further erosion.

All parts of coltsfoot are edible and can be wildcrafted for tea. However, because plant parts emerge at different times, they must be wildcrafted separately. In the early spring, wildcraft flowers and stalks and dry them to use later; harvest the leaves later in the spring and the roots in the fall.

Use shears or pruners to harvest aerial parts and a hand trowel to collect the roots, taking care to wildcraft only a small amount of roots from each plant to avoid killing the plant. All parts of the plant can be cleaned and dried in a dehydrator or on a screen, and then stored in an airtight container for future use.

Medicinal Uses

Boil the plant material in hot water, covered, to make a strong tea. Other herbs such as garlic, ground ivy, onion, mints, and mullein (because of the fine hairs on mullein, strain the tea through a coffee filter before drinking it) can also be added to the tea to support lung health. Strain the tea and sweeten it with honey before enjoying it hot. You can also prepare an infusion as a syrup mixed with other lung herbs such as horehound, mullein, and wild cherry bark.

Future Harvests

Coltsfoot is a resilient plant that spreads easily. It is deemed noxious by gardeners and farmers in some areas. Nevertheless, harvest the plant with regard to its availability in the area to help ensure its sustainability.

Cautions, Concerns, and Considerations

Like borage and comfrey, coltsfoot contains alkaloids which research has found to cause liver damage when consumed in high concentrations. Use this herb only with supervision by a trained practitioner.

HERBAL PREPARATIONS

Coltsfoot tea
Decoction
Drink ¼ cup as needed.

---

comfrey

Symphytum officinale
boneset, knitbone
PARTS USED flowers, leaves, stalks

*As a reputable tissue- and wound-healer, comfrey is an
important plant for the apothecary and first aid kit.*

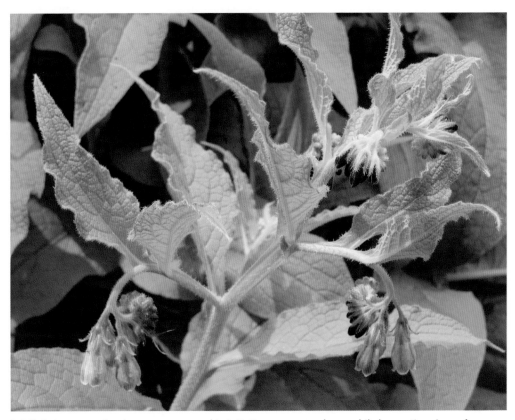

Bristly hairs on comfrey leaves can cause skin irritations, so wear gloves while harvesting. A comfrey
soak, compress, or wash can be beneficial in wound healing, or in the event of a break or soft tissue
damage.

How to Identify

Comfrey is a rapidly growing perennial that thrives in well-drained and nutrient-rich soil. First leaves emerge in early spring, and the plant sends up a stalk of 2–3 feet in mid-spring. Leaves are ovate, simple, and covered in hairs; they can be up to 10 inches long, growing alternately along the hairy stem. Comfrey flowers in late spring with racemes of symmetrical and tubular blooms that range in color from white to purple.

Botanicals for Chapped Cheeks

Many products line the pharmacy shelves, claiming to heal dry skin and protect it from chafing and chapping. Conventional products often contain synthetic chemicals derived from petroleum, and although they may act like sealants on the epidermis, or outer portion of the skin, they do little to heal the dermis, the layer below the epidermis that contains blood vessels, lymph vessels, hair follicles, and sweat glands.

Create a batch of chapped-cheek balm in your kitchen using just three ingredients: beeswax, herbs, and olive oil. Beeswax helps solidify the balm and works as a protective layer on the skin without leaving a greasy feeling.

Apply the balm before heading outside to protect your skin from harsh elements. If your skin feels sensitive in the shower, apply the balm before you rinse off. This will protect your skin from overdrying, and the hot water will help the botanicals soak deep into the dermis for healing.

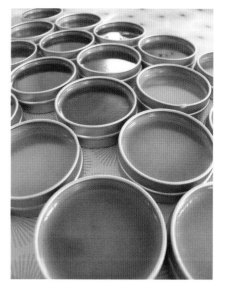

It is easy to make your own healing salve using wild plants such as calendula, chickweed, comfrey, and plantain. These deep tissue–healers can repair cracks and splits in the skin.

Where, When, and How to Wildcraft

Comfrey is often grown in herbalists' gardens, but the plant also grows wild in open fields and around old homesteads. Wildcraft fresh leaves in early spring before the plant goes to flower, or harvest the entire stalk, including flowers and leaves, in mid- to late spring. Hang bundles of plants to dry and store the herbs for later use. When harvesting, wear gloves, because the bristly hairs on the leaves can irritate your skin.

Medicinal Uses

Comfrey is one of the primary herbs used for healing wounded tissues or broken bones. It is particularly helpful as a wound begins to heal. The timing in which this herb is used and the dosage are very important: using it too soon and too much could result in the wound or break healing too rapidly, causing superficial healing and raising the risk for infection, specifically with a puncture wound or abrasion.

Comfrey can also be taken internally as a tea as part of a wound-healing protocol, in combination with other nourishing herbs such as horsetail, nettle, oatstraw, and red clover.

A comfrey soak, compress, or wash can help heal wounds, breaks, or soft tissue damage (such as sprains or torn ligaments or tendons). Comfrey infused in castor oil works wonderfully as massage oil. It's also an excellent ingredient in a basic gardener's skin-healing salve, along with chickweed, goldenrod, plantain, St. John's wort, and yarrow.

Future Harvests

Comfrey grows with wild abandon and will take over large portions of garden or wild space. Harvesting it will help control its growth. It is easily transplanted by root cuttings to grow in containers.

Cautions, Concerns, and Considerations

There is a great deal of discussion in the herbal community regarding the safety of comfrey, based on the presence of alkaloids which research has found to cause liver damage when consumed in high concentrations. It is always prudent, if in doubt, to choose to work with another herb.

Another concern is the issue of overhealing tissues or wounds with superficial use of comfrey. This has been substantiated, and comfrey is known to cause significant problems if it is used in large quantities, resulting in a wound that will not heal fully or that seals in infection.

Comfrey can also encourage production of scar tissue, which can inhibit circulation and healthy movements in the long term. When using comfrey, closely monitor the healing process, and if there are signs of overhealing or infection, discontinue its use immediately.

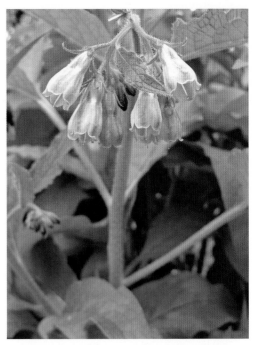

Comfrey is one of the primary herbs for tissue healing in the repair of a wound, soft tissue damage, or bone break.

HERBAL PREPARATIONS

Comfrey tea
Decoction
Drink ¼ cup as needed, or use externally as a compress, wash, or soak.

Comfrey-infused oil
1 part fresh leaves, chopped
2 parts oil
or
1 part dry leaves, chopped
4 parts oil
Use for massage.

cottonwood

Populus species

eastern cottonwood (*P. deltoides*), black cottonwood (*P. balsamifera*), big-tooth aspen (*P. grandidentata*)

PARTS USED buds, twigs

The resinous, aromatic, and spicy buds of the cottonwood can be used in an excellent muscle rub salve or liniment that's great for soothing sports injuries or tense muscles.

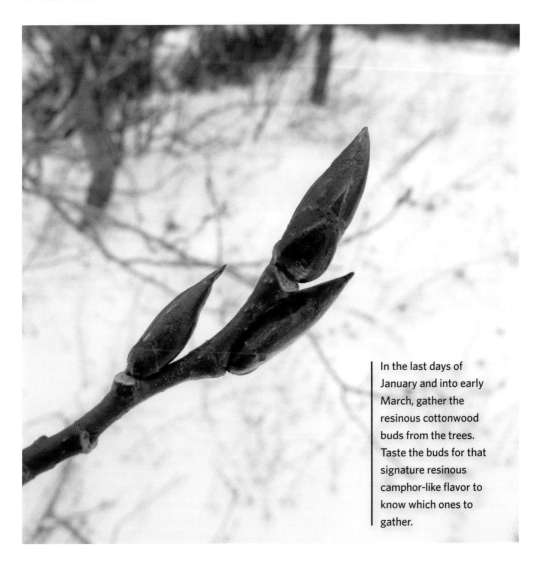

In the last days of January and into early March, gather the resinous cottonwood buds from the trees. Taste the buds for that signature resinous camphor-like flavor to know which ones to gather.

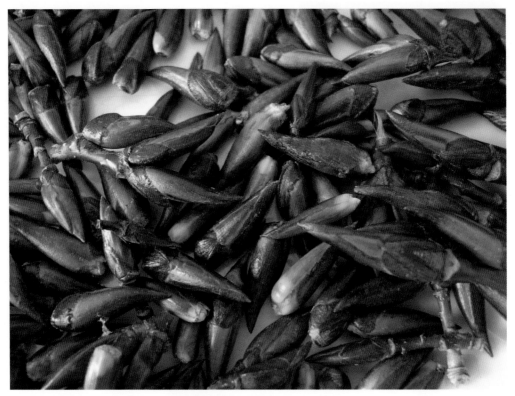

A bounty of resinous, aromatic cottonwood buds. Use the spicy buds in formulations with goldenrod, St. John's wort, and yarrow for a well-rounded infused oil, tincture, or topical liniment.

How to Identify

Cottonwoods and poplars are common along riverbanks and at water's edge, and many species grow to heights of 65–150 feet at maturity.

Eastern cottonwood, *P. deltoides*, has grayish bark, yellow twigs, and triangular, toothed leaves of about 4–6 inches long.

Black cottonwood, *P. balsamifera*, has greenish gray bark and flat leaves that are more ovate and slightly smaller, at 3–6 inches long.

Big-tooth aspen, *P. grandidentata*, has gray-green bark with horizontal lenticels. Leaves are triangular in shape, 3–4 inches long, with flat petioles. Male and female catkins bloom in late spring.

Various *Populus* species have resinous buds that are used medicinally, though they vary in degree of resin and flavor. It is common for one species of *Populus* to undergo hybridization with trees of other species in the genus.

Where, When, and How to Wildcraft

Look for cottonwood trees growing near wetlands and riverbeds, or anywhere that maintains a moist environment. From the last days of January to early March, gather the buds from the trees. Taste the buds for their signature resinous, camphor-like flavor to determine the best ones to gather. The flavor can vary from tree to tree, species to species, and locale to locale. Use your senses to determine strength and how you might want to use them.

Gather twigs in the early spring. Process buds into an oil infusion or twigs into tincture soon after harvesting to ensure the most benefits from the resin.

Medicinal Uses

Buds can be extracted in a coconut or olive oil base to create a balm of Gilead muscle salve. Buds can also be extracted as a tincture in high-proof alcohol to create a topical liniment for tight and sore muscles. Buds work well in formulations with goldenrod, St. John's wort, and yarrow for a well-rounded muscle salve or liniment.

Future Harvests

Cottonwoods may drop branches during heavy windstorms, and gathering twigs and buds from fallen branches is the most sustainable way to wildcraft. If you gather buds from live trees, take only a small handful from each tree, and be sure to give thanks for the harvest the trees offer.

HERBAL PREPARATIONS

Cottonwood tincture

1 part fresh buds and twigs, chopped
2 parts menstruum (95 percent alcohol,
   5 percent distilled water)
Take 15–20 drops as needed, or use topically as a liniment.

Cottonwood-infused oil

1 part fresh buds
2 parts oil
Use for massage.

Balm of Gilead oil

1 cup fresh buds
olive or coconut oil
Add the buds to a mason jar, and cover them completely with olive or coconut oil. Let the mixture steep for 6 weeks, and then strain. Use for massage oil, or add other herbs such as goldenrod, St. John's wort, and yarrow to create a soothing salve.

crampbark

Viburnum species
guelder rose (*V. opulus*), American highbush cranberry (*V. trilobum*)
PARTS USED bark, twigs

Crampbark is an effective medicinal plant to use for relieving dull aches and cramping in the body—from women's monthly cramping to spasmodic muscular and skeletal pain.

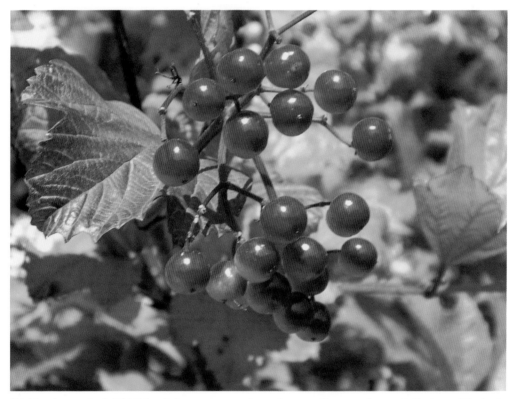

Bright red crampbark (*V. trilobum*) drupes are easy to spot among the green leaves. A tincture of the bark and twigs can be used topically as a liniment, and the fresh bark can be extracted to make a massage oil or salve.

How to Identify

This deciduous shrub grows 10–12 feet in height, with dense and spreading branches and thin, gray bark that smells skunky when scratched. Leaves are bright green and lobed—they resemble maple leaves in shape—with silvery undersides, arranged oppositely along the branches.

Flowers open from late spring to early summer and are arranged in showy white corymbs of about 3–4 inches in diameter, with fertile flowers on the inside, rimmed by sterile flowers on the outer edges. In the fall, *V. trilobum* produces berries, or drupes, of edible, tart, and slightly acidic red fruits. The drupes of *V. opulus* are unpleasantly bitter and inedible. Also in the fall, the foliage begins to change color to beautiful hues of reds and yellows.

Where, When, and How to Wildcraft

Crampbark prefers moist and nutrient-rich soil, but it tolerates a variety of soil pH levels. Look for it growing along the edges of fields and woodlands; it's also a common cultivated garden shrub. In the early spring before the plant leafs out, prune back the exterior branches. Strip the branches of the thin, gray bark and branch tips and process these into oil or tincture, or dry them to use later for tea.

Both *V. opulus* and *V. trilobum* can be used interchangeably; however, some herbalists note some slight variations in their ability to soothe cramping. To taste relaxant strength, seek out the aroma and flavor of the bark: the more skunky the aroma, the stronger the relaxant nature of the plant.

Medicinal Uses

Use a tincture of crampbark topically as a liniment massaged over cramping areas or internally to help soothe spasmodic pain. Extract the fresh bark in oil to create massage oil or salve to soothe cramping pains.

Extracting crampbark into castor oil makes a doubly soothing lymphatic massage oil good for uterine menstrual contractions or spasmodic pain associated with urinary tract infections or kidney stones.

Future Harvests

Crampbark is a common shrub, and removing the bark from pruned branches in early spring will not significantly affect future harvests.

HERBAL PREPARATIONS

Crampbark tea
Decoction
Drink ¼ cup as needed, or use externally as a hot compress.

Crampbark tincture
1 part fresh bark and twigs, chopped
2 parts menstruum (95 percent alcohol,
   5 percent distilled water)
or
1 part dry bark and twigs, chopped
4 parts menstruum (95 percent alcohol,
5 percent distilled water)
Take 25 drops as needed.

Crampbark-infused oil
1 part fresh bark and twigs, chopped
2 parts oil
Use for massage.

---

cranberry

Vaccinium species
small cranberry (*V. oxycoccos*), large cranberry (*V. macrocarpon*)
PARTS USED fruit

Cranberries are high in antioxidants and vitamins. A functional food and astringent herbal remedy, wild cranberry medicine helps support healthy urinary tract function.

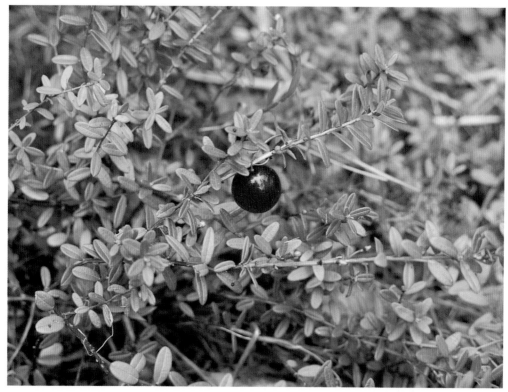

Cranberry shrubs produce harvestable fruit in their second year. Cranberry preparations are useful in the treatment of recurrent urinary tract infections.

How to Identify

Wild cranberry is a small evergreen vining shrub that can spread across rocky outcrops and low-lying vegetation. Scraggly, woody branches grow up to 12 inches long and spread across the ground, creating a mat of leaves and small branches dotted with berries. Its dark green leaves are small, from ½ inch (small cranberry) to 1 inch (large cranberry) long, and ovate, and they are arranged alternately along greenish red stems. Leaf margins curl under.

Flowers vary in color from white to pink; they appear singly at the end of a long stalk.

Small fruits are ready to harvest in fall and winter.

Where, When, and How to Wildcraft

Look for cranberries growing low to the ground along sandy lake shores, in bogs, and in wetlands. Because bogs are pretty magical places, you should make harvest day an adventure; pack a picnic to enjoy the experience.

Harvest the small, red or dark pink berries in the fall and winter. The plant goes dormant after its first year until the following summer, when the fruit develops. The berries overwinter well and can even be discovered on winter hikes in places where the snow has blown away. Gather berries by hand into baskets. Cranberries are tedious to pick by hand, but they are worth the effort; high in nutrient content, they store well refrigerated or dried.

If the vines are clear of other vegetation, you can use a hand rake to gather the berries and quicken harvest time—this method, however, will also gather unwanted leaves and plant material that you must remove later. Firm, clean, and dry cranberries can be stored for many months in dry cloth market bags in the bottom of the refrigerator or in cold storage through the winter. Cranberries can also be dried in a dehydrator. Press fresh berries for juice and use dry berries for tea.

Medicinal Uses

Preparations of cranberry are beneficial in instances of recurrent urinary tract infections. As a functional food, cranberry juice is a low-sugar beverage, and its astringency can help tighten and tone the urinary tissues, making them less susceptible to infection.

A tincture of cranberry fruit can also be part of a urinary tract protocol that may include echinacea (if infection is present),

goldenrod, plantain (for tissue repair and healing), and wild yam (for cramping and spasmodic pain).

Future Harvests

The biggest threat to the wild cranberry isn't overharvesting, but the rapid rate at which wetlands and bogs are disappearing across the upper Midwest to development, as well as upstream watershed pollution and contamination. A bog is a special place, and each plant medicine-maker should do his or her part to help protect and preserve these fragile ecosystems.

HERBAL PREPARATIONS

Cranberry tea
Decoction
Drink 1 cup, 3 times per day for acute infection.

Cranberry tincture
1 part fresh berries
2 parts menstruum (50 percent alcohol, 50 percent distilled water)
Take 10–25 drops for an acute infection.

---

dandelion

Taraxacum officinale

PARTS USED flowers, leaves, roots

*The dastardly dandelion is much more than a weed and a salad green. Its flow-
ers, leaves, and roots are useful to support digestion, the lymphatic system, and
healthy urinary tract function. It is a perfect medicine that's readily available
and easy to find.*

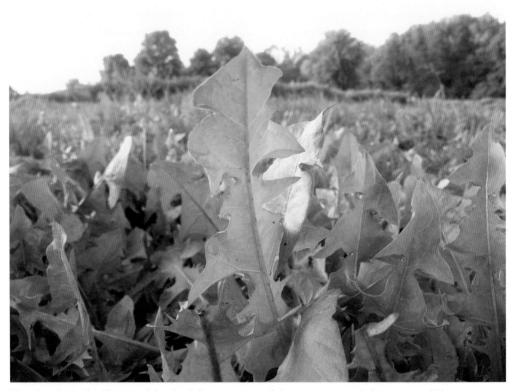

The sharply toothed leaves of the dandelion are some of the spring season's first green edibles.

How to Identify

Spiky dandelion leaves emerge from the
white root crown in a basal rosette, followed
by several smooth, hollow 3- to 4-inch flower
stalks. The flowers of the dandelion are familiar—yellow, flat-topped, and cupped by small,
green, pointed bracts that turn upward and
close the flower when rain is imminent.

Root size and girth are dependent on
the soil: roots are more substantial in well-
drained, composted soil and smaller in dry,
rocky, nutrient-deficient earth.

Where, When, and How to Wildcraft

Dandelions grow almost everywhere and are
easy to find. In early spring when the weather

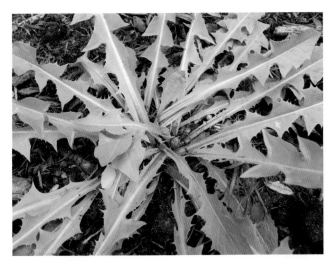
Rosettes of dandelion leaves are familiar sights in urban yards.

Medicinal Uses

Dandelion root is a helpful metabolic tonic for the digestive system, where it aids in digestion and absorption of minerals. Roast the root and prepare it in a tea or tincture to include as part of a digestive herbal blend. Dandelion root tea has an affinity for the urinary tract system and can be included as part of a protocol to support healthy urinary function when mixed with other plants such as cranberry and echinacea.

is cool and moist, the rapidly growing leaves will be most tender and choice for eating raw. The leaves are again tender and delicious in cool fall weather. Harvest the leaves with garden shears or by hand and gently clean them in the kitchen. Leaves are best when picked in the early morning.

In midspring, as the weather warms, pluck the flowers easily with your fingers. Because they are difficult to wash well, harvest flowers that are free from significant dust and debris.

Dandelions that grow in the shade will be more tender and sweet than those growing in direct sun. They will also bloom later. Leaves become significantly more bitter, dry, and rough after the dandelion goes to flower and seed and as the weather becomes warm in summer.

Dig the roots any time across the seasons. The soil quality and moisture determine whether the roots will be easy or difficult to remove. Use a hand-digging tool, and be careful not to break off the taproot midway. Both the crowns and roots will need a good brushing and scrubbing in the kitchen to remove excess soil.

As a lymphatic herb, dandelion flowers can be used in a topical oil to massage over cystic and fibrous tissues. I like to use a dandelion flower oil massage to bring sunshine and vibrancy to tissues that may be stagnant and stuck, particularly the lymphatic breast and pectoral tissues below the armpits and the tender lymphatic tissues along the leg and groin regions.

Dandelion flower–infused oil works well with infused oils of calendula, plantain, and violet flowers and leaves. This gentle herbal infusion is helpful for Maya abdominal massage. (This well-known technique was developed by naturopath Rosita Arvigo, based on her apprenticeship with Mayan healer Don Elijio Panti.) It can also be used as a massage oil for postpartum mothers.

Dandelion should also be included regularly at the dinner table. Bitter greens such as dandelion help the stomach in digestion by increasing bile production. It's a good spring habit to add handfuls of wild leaves to meals a few times a day, if possible.

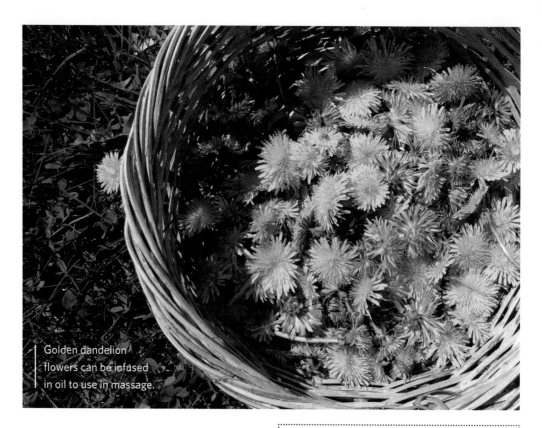
Golden dandelion flowers can be infused in oil to use in massage.

Future Harvests

Its nutrition, versatility, and abundance makes dandelion such an amazing plant medicine that it never ceases to amaze me why homeowners everywhere don't let these plants take over their lawns. Dandelion is truly a wildly free medicinal!

HERBAL PREPARATIONS

Dandelion root tea
Decoction
Drink ¼ cup, 3 times per day.

Dandelion root tincture
1 part fresh roots, chopped
2 parts menstruum (50 percent alcohol, 50 percent distilled water)
or
1 part dry roots, chopped
4 parts menstruum (50 percent alcohol, 50 percent distilled water)
Take 25–30 drops per day.

Dandelion flower–infused oil
1 part fresh flowers
2 parts oil
Use for massage.

Rumex species
sorrel
PARTS USED leaves, roots, seeds

Dock helps with digestion and is rich in minerals and nutrients, with high amounts of vitamins A and C. It can also help support a healthy metabolism.

How to Identify
Perennial dock is easy to identify. The cold-tolerant leaves emerge in early spring with straight, wavy, or curly edges, growing from 3 to 12 inches long. In midsummer,

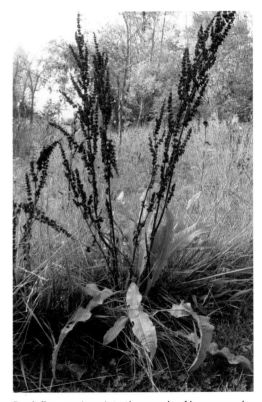

Dock flowers ripen into thousands of brown seeds on tall spikes. As a mineral supplement, dock root can be used to create a mineral-dense syrup for iron deficiency or to support digestion with other herbs as part of a bitters formula.

dock sends up flower stalks up to 5 feet tall that bear small whorls of green or dark red flowers. These tiny flowers ripen by late summer into thousands of brown, winged seeds.

Dock roots are substantial, especially in nutrient-rich soil, and range in color from creamy white to yellow. The entire plant is predominantly bitter in flavor.

Where, When, and How to Wildcraft
Dock is abundant and grows wildly in empty lots and fields. Look for it in early spring when the leaves are tender and choice. Leaves become tough and relatively uninteresting in flavor as the plant blooms and the weather becomes warm.

Flowers bloom in late spring. In summer, stalks are topped with dense, brown clusters of seeds in open fields among the evening primrose, blue chicory, and the tall but not yet flowering goldenrod. Gather seeds in late summer or early fall after they have dried on the stalks. In the kitchen, dry them completely in a dehydrator before storing.

Gather roots in fall after the plant has gone to seed. Clean the roots and store them for up to several weeks in the refrigerator.

Medicinal Uses
Dock root is particularly high in iron and can be used to create a mineral-dense molasses syrup. Decoct the root in water, reduce the liquid in volume to one-third, and then strain

it before preserving it with equal amounts of black-strap molasses. Heating the mixture extracts the roots' minerals into the decoction. Use this syrup as you would health food store preparations at a fraction of the cost.

To support digestion, blend the root tincture with carminative herbs (spicebush, sarsaparilla, lemon balm, or cinnamon) and burdock root to help strengthen the digestion and assimilation of nutrients.

Incorporate dock leaves into cooking to help with digestion. Leaves are nutrient rich, with high amounts of vitamins A and C.

Dock seeds are protein-dense. For those interested in athletic performance, add the seeds to a wild granola of amaranth, chia, and wild nuts for a boost of plant protein.

Future Harvests

Dock reproduces by self-seeding prolifically. You can help it flourish by sharing the seed harvest with wildlife and by scattering seeds as you head back to the kitchen.

Cautions, Concerns, and Considerations

Because dock takes up a significant amount of minerals into its roots, leaves, and stalks, be careful where you harvest and make sure the soil is free of lead or other heavy metal contamination.

HERBAL PREPARATIONS

Dock tea
Decoction
Drink ¼ cup per day.

Dock root tincture
1 part fresh roots, chopped
2 parts menstruum (50 percent alcohol, 50 percent distilled water)
or
1 part dry roots, chopped
4 parts menstruum (50 percent alcohol, 50 percent distilled water)
Take 15 drops as needed.

eastern white cedar

Thuja occidentalis
American arborvitae, white cedar
PARTS USED leaves

Use the aromatic leaves of eastern white cedar to make a warming tea or astringent skin wash. Their astringent nature makes them helpful for sinus issues as well.

How to Identify
This evergreen grows in woodland areas to varying heights, from a shrub to a tree up to 30 feet tall. Its wood is soft and pliable. Bark is dark brownish red, scaly, and furrowed, and it peels away from the trunk in long strips. The dark green fans of flat leaves are textured, scaly, and about 1½ to 2 inches long. Small brown cones begin to take shape in early summer and grow into fully formed clusters by late fall.

Where, When, and How to Wildcraft
Look for eastern white cedar in woodlands, swamps, and along the sandy cliffs of the Great Lakes. This fast-growing native and ornamental hardwood grows throughout the northern parts of the Midwest. It tolerates the damp soils of cedar swamps and is common in landscape plantings. Gather leaves from live or wind-fallen branches in any season.

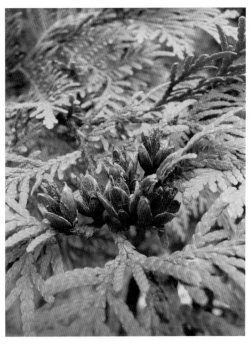

Eastern white cedar's aromatic leaves make a warming tea, astringent skin wash, and ceremonial smudge stick.

Medicinal Uses
An herbal steam or tea that includes the aromatic leaves is useful for clearing the sinuses. The tea is astringent and drying and can help move respiratory congestion. The aromatics of the tea or tincture also soothe digestion. Add honey to sweeten.

As a topical wash, tea made from the eastern white cedar leaves can help astringe and clear up topical infections. In an oil infusion, its leaves are used in protocols for healing various skin melanomas. It works well in combination with calendula, chaga, echinacea, reishi, rose, and St. John's wort. Extract its essence in raw honey and strain it for a topical honey paste.

The eastern white cedar has long been used in traditional ceremonies, incorporated

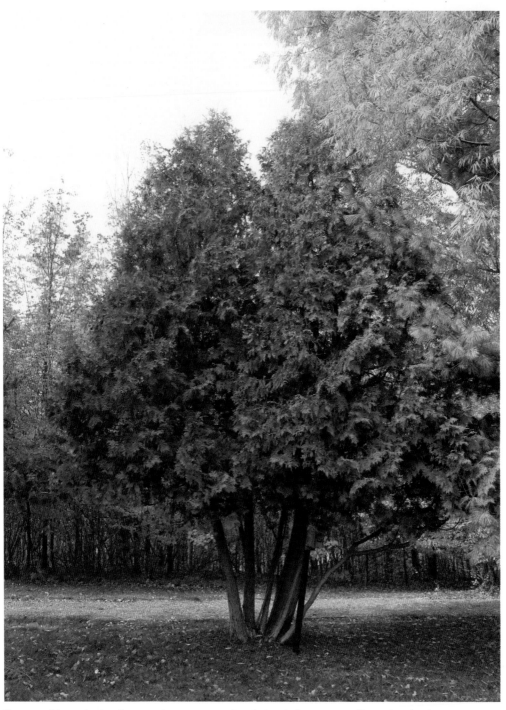

Eastern white cedar is a fast-growing evergreen that thrives in forests as well as urban landscapes.

into a smudge stick or medicine bundle. Gather it in a ceremonial way, and consider including other space-clearing herbs such as artemisia, sage, and yarrow.

Future Harvests

Avoid harvesting from old-growth cedar forests to help preserve these important habitats. Gather its leaves in moderation or from wind-fallen boughs to help preserve wild stands.

HERBAL PREPARATIONS

Eastern white cedar tea
Infusion
Drink ¼ cup, or use externally as an astringent skin wash.

Eastern white cedar tincture
1 part fresh leaves, chopped
2 parts menstruum (50 percent alcohol, 50 percent distilled water)
Take 10–15 drops as needed.

Eastern white cedar–infused oil
1 part fresh leaves, chopped
2 parts oil
Use for massage.

echinacea

Echinacea species
prairie doctor, purple coneflower
PARTS USED aerial parts, roots

Echinacea stimulates the immune system and helps clear systemic septic and topical infections. It also assists the body in fighting off viruses and illness.

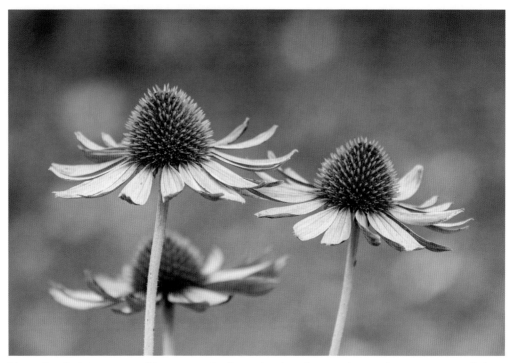

The entire plant, from root to blossom, can be dug and gathered across the growing season as needed. The aerial parts can also be simply gathered with garden clippers, bound, and dried for later use.

How to Identify

Echinacea is a perennial native wildflower with coarse and hairy, dark green, lance-shaped leaves. Stalks of 18–36 inches bear flowers from early summer to fall. Echinacea flowers are inflorescences—collections of 200–300 small fertile florets bunched together on a cone. Each brownish orange cone-shaped head of stiff and spikey flowers is surrounded by petal-like florets, which range in color from light pink to a deep and vibrant fuchsia or purple.

Where, When, and How to Wildcraft

Look for this native perennial in sunny spots in open fields. It often escapes from gardens and naturalizes in surrounding areas. Harvest the entire plant, from roots to blossoms, throughout the growing season as needed. Dig the roots with a spade. Harvest the stalks

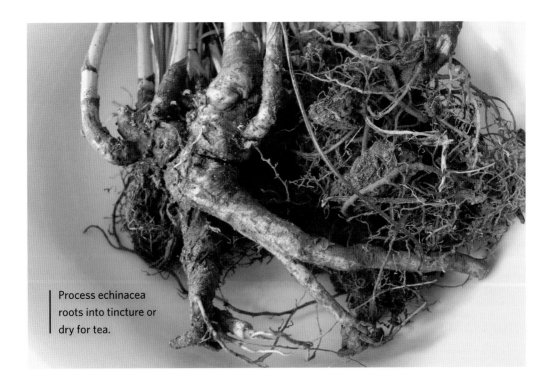

Process echinacea roots into tincture or dry for tea.

and bind and hang them to dry for later use. Store plant materials when completely dry in airtight containers.

Medicinal Uses

Echinacea is not a culinary herb but is most commonly known as an herbal remedy to use at the onset of colds and flus to help boost immunity and assist the body in fighting off viruses and illness. The entire plant (roots to flowers) can be dried for use in tea or tinctured in alcohol.

To use echinacea as an immunity booster, consume it as tea or plant extract tincture at the first symptoms of a cold or flu. Combine echinacea with elderberry to help increase the immune system's response to a virus.

Echinacea also helps clear systemic and topical infections. With an infection such as mastitis, use a tincture of echinacea in combination with ceanothus and poke root tinctures to help clear the stuck duct and ease the infection. Use echinacea tea as a topical wash to clean wounds and help prevent infection. Add echinacea tea to the bath for a systemic approach to soothing a poison ivy infection.

Dried echinacea quickly loses its potency. One way to test for potency is to taste the dried plant material and wait for a distinct "zing" on your tongue. It should make your mouth tingle and incite a desire to spit. You will find that the echinacea you harvest and dry will be leaps and bounds better in quality than any echinacea you purchase, with harvest dates unknown and vitality lacking.

Future Harvests

To preserve and sustain the plant populations, it's best to gather echinacea from established plant communities. But in a pinch, you can also harvest and use younger and smaller echinacea plants effectively.

Loss of prairie habitat has greatly affected the distribution of *Echinacea angustifolia* in the

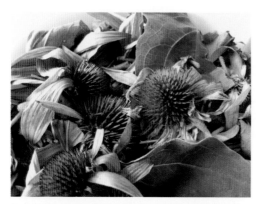

Dry the harvested fresh leaves and flowers of echinacea for tea blends.

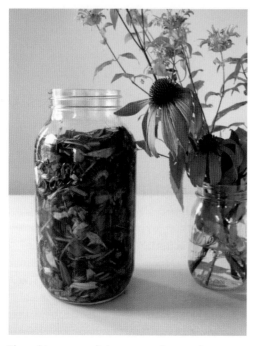

The echinacea medicines you make—such as a root, leaf, and flower tincture—will be far superior to commercially available products.

wild. It isn't as common as it once was, and the majority of the available echinacea today is *E. purpurea*. Your support of habitat preservation and cultivation of native wildflowers will help sustain this attractive medicinal herb. It can be propagated by seed or transplants in the garden.

Cautions, Concerns, and Considerations

Remember that echinacea is not a replacement for rest, healthy food, and sleep, which are needed to promote the body's core immunity. Echinacea and other immune-boosting herbs such as boneset, elderberry, and yarrow should not be used as a replacement for these foundational components of wellness.

HERBAL PREPARATIONS

Echinacea tea
Decoction
Drink 1 cup, 3 to 5 times per day, or use externally as a skin wash.

Echinacea tincture
1 part fresh flowers, leaves, and roots, chopped
2 parts menstruum (50 percent alcohol, 50 percent distilled water)
or
1 part dry flowers, leaves, and roots, chopped
4 parts menstruum (50 percent alcohol, 50 percent distilled water)
Take 25–30 drops, 3 to 5 times per day for infection.

Sambucus nigra
black elder, European elderberry
PARTS USED berries, flowers

Elderflowers and elderberries are useful in herbal remedies to fight off colds, flus, and other viruses. The flowers are delicious in a honey infusion, and the berries can be used to make a syrup that's chock-full of antioxidants to add to cocktails or use as a base for a traditional vinegar-and-honey shrub.

How to Identify
Elder is a large deciduous shrub or small tree 20 feet tall and wide at maturity. Its bark is light gray and furrowed, and its wood is brittle. Branches are hollow with a pithy inner core.

Elder leaves are arranged in opposite pairs, pinnate, with five to seven lance-shaped leaflets that are smooth, toothed, and 2–6 inches long. In midsummer, the elder's fragrant white flowers unfold in terminal clusters on showy umbels. The first of the elderflowers open after summer solstice in June, and blooms continue through mid-July. Fresh elderflowers have a fragrant, citrusy scent.

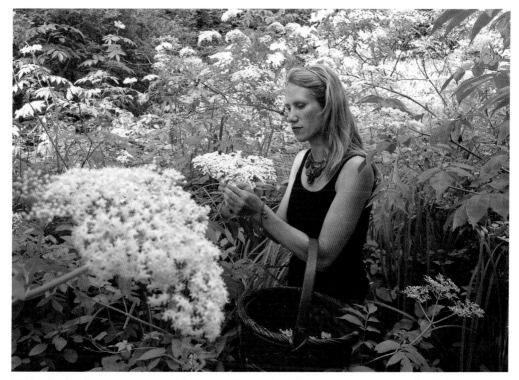

Wildcraft elderflowers to use as a relaxant tea for treating a fever or promoting a good night's rest.

Crafting a Cold and Flu Game Plan

It's unavoidable. Being human means we will get the icky sniffles at some point this winter season, but the good news is that our bodies are amazingly designed with built-in immune responses to defend against viral or bacterial infections. The trick is working with these immune system responses to ensure that we can defend against further debility and return to everyday life just as strong as before.

Consider this general game-plan before you start to get sick so you can choose helpful therapeutics, recover, and get back to the game of life more quickly.

- Recognize the early warning signs. Stressed? Feeling worn out? Aches? Pains? These may be early signals from your body telling you to slow down. If you are under excess stress, you are more susceptible to illness. Dial back and rest, and you will be able to negotiate the coming weeks without illness. Nourish your body with good food, sleep, and vitamin D.
- When you first start feeling sick, try to kick the ick early and use herbal therapeutics to support your body's immune processes. Bust out the elderberry syrup, which can help inhibit a virus's ability to reproduce. Echinacea also can help boost the peripheral immune system. Herbal combination teas such as elderflower, mint, and yarrow are a must-have for the beginnings of a cold or flu, to stimulate the immune system and relax the body.
- Set your work aside, get some rest, and get better quicker. Renegotiate any short-term commitments to allow for some significant rest. I know this is difficult for us parents or for folks with work schedules that aren't very flexible. Do what you can to rearrange the workload so your immune system gets some space to fight the infection. Remember that energy put into work while you are sick is energy that could be used for healing. And the potential cost of pushing through a cold or flu virus is a secondary bacterial infection. No one wants that.
- Got a fever? Don't try suppressing natural immune responses. Remember that fevers are not illnesses; they are ways the body helps fight illness. They are on your team!
- Support a fever's therapeutic actions with herbs such as boneset, chamomile,

The shrub begins bearing clusters of fruit when it reaches about 5 feet tall. The deep purple and black berries usually ripen in mid- to late August.

Where, When, and How to Wildcraft

Look for elder growing in hedgerows, along edges of fields, and in drainage ditches and other low-lying areas where water flows.

Gather elderflowers by cutting the umbels from the shrub, taking care to gather only the open blossoms. Use large baskets or boxes to hold the umbels so they are not crushed, and lay them flat on a screen to dry. Separate the dry flowers from the stems and store them for later use.

In mid- to late August, gather only the umbels with dark purple to black berries that elderflower, ginger, mints, and yarrow. These are wonderful when used for hot teas (and the hot water is a therapy itself). These herbs will help the body produce an effective fever and also help relax the body and soothe aches and pains.

- For those sniffles, work with the body's attempts at trying to loosen and move phlegm and mucus to restore healthy tone to the respiratory tissues. Using an over-the-counter mucus eliminator is counterintuitive to maintaining healthy tissues—mucus is good!
- Soothe the congestion. Try an aromatic herbal steam inhalation with mints, pine needles, and sage in a pot of hot water to open the sinuses. Eat onion and garlic in copious amounts for their antimicrobial benefits. Raw honey is also helpful, especially for soothing a dry cough. A relaxant lung herb such as cherry bark or mullein can help open the lungs, and elecampane can help with damp, wet coughs (it's helpful for bacterial infections, too).
- Don't forget the chicken soup. Hot, nourishing, clear broths prepared with cayenne, garlic, and onions will help warm the body, and the aromatic kitchen herbs help clear clogged sinuses and offer antimicrobial benefits.
- Clean out the gunk. Rest. Repeat. As your body starts to feel better, your lymphatic system will be working to clean up the debris left over from your immune system's battle. Support this lymphatic work by consuming liquids and broths, plus teas or tinctures made with herbs such as ceanothus or mullein—or simply add lemon to hot water. This will help move the gunk from your body as it returns to normal.
- Don't jump back into the grind the first moment you feel better. Continue to take it easy for ten days or so after a serious illness. Slowly reintroduce work, stresses, and strenuous physical activities over time. This will all help prevent a secondary bacterial infection that can easily settle in if your defenses are down and you carelessly reenter the fray.
- Once you are better, keep feeding your body good foods, and get enough sleep and exercise—these are foundational for winter wellness.
- My final advice: if you feel that your illness is beyond your control and you find yourself turning to Google for answers, see a doctor.

are free of dust and bird droppings. The berries don't need to be washed; in fact, washing can actually damage very ripe, juicy berries. In the kitchen, wild-harvested berries are often hosts to hitchhiking spiders that were hiding among the fruit (although I find this less of a nuisance and more a part of its magic).

Before freezing or drying berries, separate them from the stems which you should discard; consuming the stems may cause stomach upset.

Medicinal Uses

Use dry or fresh elderflowers in a delightful tea that performs as a relaxant. It will incite a bit of sweating when enjoyed hot. Because of this, elderflower is commonly used for colds and flu to support a productive fever and

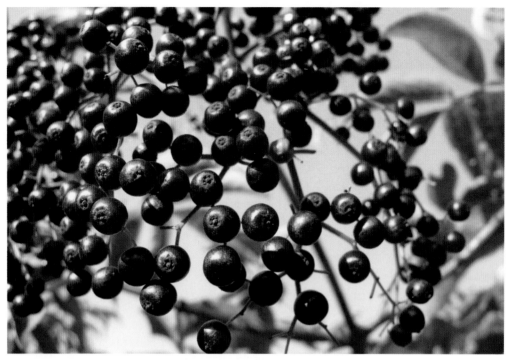

Elderberries ripen in late summer and are quickly devoured by birds. Elderberry is filled with antioxidants and flavonoids that stimulate the body's inflammation response.

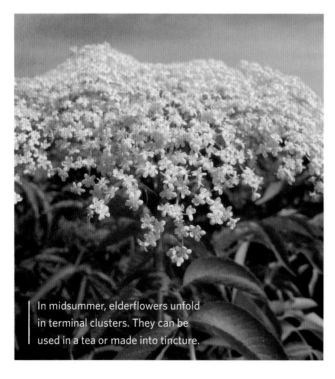

In midsummer, elderflowers unfold in terminal clusters. They can be used in a tea or made into tincture.

relax tension from body aches.

Elderflower makes such a sweetly mild tea that children easily take to sipping it, especially if they are under the weather. It mixes well with peppermint and a bit of yarrow, in a classic gypsy tea recipe. Elderflower tea is also nice sipped in the evening as a way to relax and prepare for bedtime.

You can also make homemade elderberry syrup with neutral grain spirits and raw honey. Not only is it more delicious than commercially available products, but homemade elderberry syrup is much more affordable. Consider adding boneset, catnip, spotted bee balm, wild

Cold and Flu First Responder: Elderberry

Plant medicines such as elderberry can help shorten the lifespan of a virus—if you know when and how to use them. Medical research shows that if you heed your body's warnings and take preparations of elderberry elixir within the first 48 hours of the start of a virus, the symptoms experienced with colds and flus can be decreased by as much as four days.

How does elderberry work? It is not only filled with useful antioxidants and flavonoids, but it stimulates the body's inflammation response against the virus, which then inhibits the virus's ability to reproduce.

bergamot, and yarrow for an herb-fortified elderberry elixir. The flavor of elderflower is light and works well with other flavors that are equally light and not overpowering.

Future Harvests

The fast-growing elder is easily propagated by cuttings. Remember, however, that the elderflowers you harvest now will mean fewer berries later. So balance out your harvest, particularly if elder isn't prolific in your area.

HERBAL PREPARATIONS

Elderflower tea
Infusion
Drink 1 cup.

Elderflower tincture
1 part fresh flowers, chopped
2 parts menstruum (50 percent alcohol,
   50 percent distilled water)
Take 25 drops as needed.

Elderberry tincture
1 part fresh berries
2 parts menstruum (50 percent alcohol,
   50 percent distilled water)
Take 25 drops as needed.

elecampane

Inula helenium

PARTS USED roots

When the lungs are full of congestion and stuck mucus, elecampane is a helpful remedy. With a flavor similar to that of camphor, elecampane can help you expectorate to dry up respiratory infections.

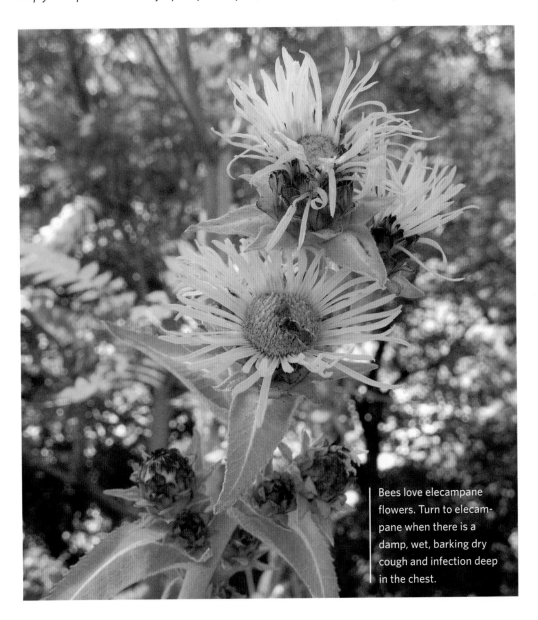

Bees love elecampane flowers. Turn to elecampane when there is a damp, wet, barking dry cough and infection deep in the chest.

How to Identify

Elecampane is a showy perennial that grows in full sun in fertile, moist soil with good drainage. At its peak height, it is 3–5 feet tall. Large, dark green, toothed, and fuzzy ovate leaves grow from a basal rosette and up the stem in an alternate arrangement. Bright yellow flower heads are 2–3 inches in diameter, with thin petals that circle an orange-yellow center ray. The perennial root is fleshy and aromatic.

Where, When, and How to Wildcraft

Look for elecampane growing in sunny locations in fields and at the edges of woodlands. It is also an easy grower in a medicinal plant garden. Gather roots at any time for medicine-making, but this is most easily done in late fall, after the plant has flowered.

Medicinal Uses

Turn to elecampane for a damp, wet, barking cough and infection deep in the chest, to stimulate stuck and damp congestion in the respiratory system. The roots of this resinous and aromatic plant can be prepared fresh as tea, tincture, or infused honey, or they can be dried for later use.

Elecampane blends well with other respiratory medicinal plants such as mullein, sage, spotted bee balm, and wild bergamot. It is particularly delicious when extracted into raw honey with these herbs and can be swallowed by the spoonful to help soothe a sore throat.

Candy fresh roots along with fresh angelica roots to make an aromatic cough drop for chewing to open up the sinuses and ease congestion.

Elecampane has a broad antibacterial capacity and can also be used internally and topically as part of a protocol to heal secondary bacterial infections caused by streptococcus, pneumonia, and antibiotic-resistant organisms.

Future Harvests

Gather only a section of the roots to avoid damaging the plant and disturbing next year's harvest. You can also divide and transplant elecampane in the fall to help encourage future growth.

HERBAL PREPARATIONS

Elecampane root tea
Decoction
Drink ¼ cup, hot.

Elecampane tincture
1 part fresh roots, chopped
2 parts menstruum (95 percent alcohol,
  5 percent distilled water)
or
1 part dry roots, chopped
4 parts menstruum (95 percent alcohol,
  5 percent distilled water)
Take 15–20 drops as needed.

---

evening primrose

Oenothera species
PARTS USED flowers, leaves, roots

From late spring through the heat of midsummer, the yellow blooms of evening primrose joyfully offer a calming medicine for fried nerves, scratchy skin, and dry lung congestion.

How to Identify

The biennial (with a two-year lifespan) evening primrose is a showy plant.

In its first year, its leaves grow in a tight basal rosette. Bright green, lance-shaped, and toothed, they are edible and delicious. In its second year, the plant sends up a 5-foot-tall, woody, and branching stalk, with leaves arranged alternately along the stem. From late spring until late July, the plant forms terminal clusters of fragrant yellow flowers, 1–2 inches wide. The root is white, fleshy, and sometimes spindly, depending on soil quality.

Where, When, and How to Wildcraft

Look for evening primrose growing in poor quality soil and waste places, where it prefers full sun. Gather the roots in the fall of the first year of the plant before energy is sent into the stalk in the second year. Gather the leaves and flowers of the second-year plant in spring and summer when the plant blooms.

Medicinal Uses

Evening primrose is a nourishing wild edible that can help restore and tone the nervous system, wounded skin, congested and dry lungs, and the lymphatic system.

For nervous exhaustion and upset digestion due to stress, use evening primrose as a calming tea or tincture with other plant medicines such as blue vervain, lemon balm, and skullcap. Integrate it with nourishing nettle, oatstraw, and red clover for a nutrient-dense tea to strengthen the nervous system.

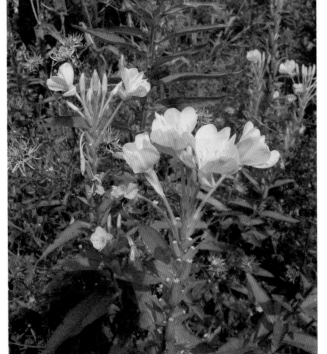

Evening primrose flowers open quickly every evening and are closed by morning, hence the plant's common name.

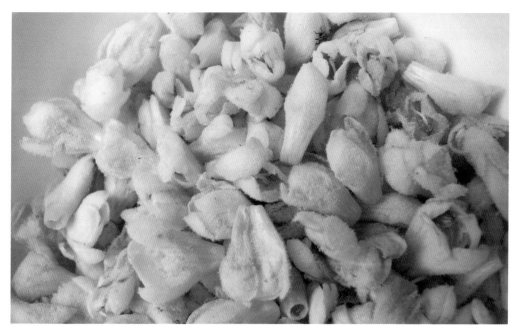
Use evening primrose flowers in teas, tinctures, and salves.

As a skin-healer, evening primrose leaves and flowers offer cooling effects when blended into a salve or a skin wash in combination with plants such as echinacea, plantain, and St. John's wort.

Like mullein flowers, evening primrose flowers have a slightly lymphatic effect. Use them in combination with dandelion flowers, mullein flowers, and violet leaves and flowers for a lymphatic tea, tincture, or massage oil blend. Flowers can also be used topically as a poultice or liniment in combination with goldenrod and mullein leaves to soothe bursitis caused by joint inflammation and trauma. Add yarrow if significant bruising is also present.

Evening primrose can help moisten and relax dryness and congestion in the lungs. Combine it with elecampane, mullein, wild cherry bark, and raw honey to make a soothing remedy to calm spasmodic coughing and promote expectoration of stuck mucus.

Future Harvests

Depending on the environment, evening primrose can grow prolifically or it can be difficult to find. Gather the roots and flowers in accordance with the plant's availability.

HERBAL PREPARATIONS

Evening primrose tea
Cold infusion
Drink 1 cup, 3 times per day, or use as an external wash.

Evening primrose tincture
1 part fresh flowers, leaves, and roots, chopped
2 parts menstruum (50 percent alcohol, 50 percent distilled water)
Take 10–15 drops as needed.

feverfew

Tanacetum parthenium
PARTS USED flowers, leaves

Use resinous and aromatic feverfew to quell a headache or skeletal tension in the neck, or include it in an herbal blend for upset digestion and fever with a cold or flu.

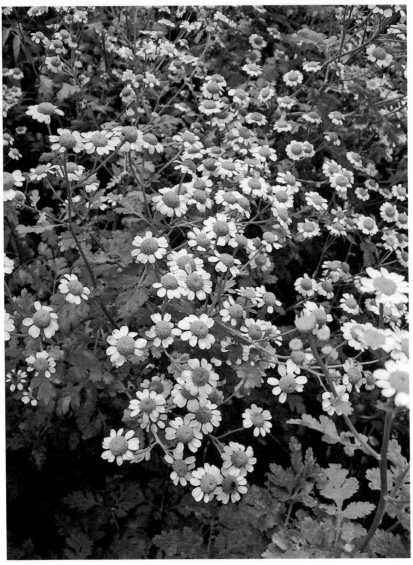

Feverfew spreads wildly in and out of the garden. Notably bitter and aromatic, it can help dispel fevers and quell headaches or nervous tension in the neck and back.

How to Identify

Feverfew is a bushy perennial herb that grows 1–2 feet tall, with bipinnate, hairy, and lobed leaves that are arranged alternately along its branching stalk. Feverfew flowers in midsummer, with small composite flowers of daisylike white rays with yellow centers. The entire plant is notably resinous and aromatic, with a distinct metallic aroma and bitter flavor.

Where, When, and How to Wildcraft

Feverfew is commonly planted in gardens, but it escapes cultivation easily and spreads wildly across disturbed soils and waste places. Gather the flowers and leaves throughout the summer while the plant is in bloom.

Medicinal Uses

Bitter and aromatic, feverfew is a helpful herb for dispelling fevers and quelling a headache or nervous tension in the neck and back. To soothe upset digestion, prepare feverfew in a tincture as part of a digestive bitters blend in combination with aspen bark and tulip poplar bark and flowers.

The bitter flavor of the plant can be a barrier to some. To make feverfew a more appetizing herb, extract it in brandy for a tincture and sweeten it slightly with raw honey for an elixir. Feverfew can also be extracted into white wine to sip in the summer.

Future Harvests

Feverfew can rapidly reproduce and spread, and because it is a perennial plant, regular gathering of the aerial parts will not affect future harvests.

HERBAL PREPARATIONS

Feverfew tea
Infusion
Drink ¼ cup.

Feverfew tincture
1 part fresh flowers and leaves, chopped
2 parts menstruum (50 percent alcohol,
  50 percent distilled water)
Take 5–10 drops as needed.

field garlic

Allium vineale
wild onion
PARTS USED bulbs, leaves

The aromatic and resinous flavors of field garlic are important and useful for the home herbalist in helping clear damp and congested lung conditions.

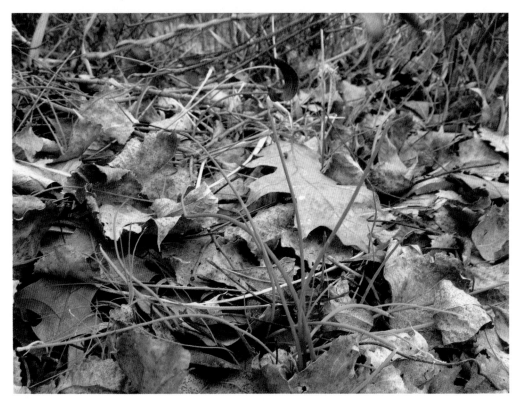

The leaves of field garlic are particularly useful for early spring colds and congestion in combination with pine needles. Sweetened with honey, this aromatic pairing can make a delicious tea to help loosen the mucosa and open the sinuses.

How to Identify

Wild field garlic is a cool-weather, clumping, perennial bulb. One of its fail-safe identifiers is its aroma, which is pungent, acrid, and garlicky. The leaves are slender hollow tubes, 12–36 inches long.

Field garlic bulbs are small, usually not larger than ¾ inch in diameter and 1 inch in length. When field garlic flowers in late spring, it produces a round head of small, purple, edible florets. It prefers cool weather and dies back in the spring, but it will return again in the fall with the rains.

Where, When, and How to Wildcraft

Look for field garlic in sun or shade in rich, well-drained soil along the edges of fields and woods and in pastures and grassy areas. It is one of the earliest spring herbs to emerge and often begins growing as the snow melts. The entire plant can be harvested and eaten, and you can wash, chop, and prepare both bulbs and leaves for use in herbal remedies.

Medicinal Uses

Because of its antimicrobial properties, field garlic can be used like conventional garlic to help with lung congestion and respiratory illnesses. Mix it into a soothing tea with mullein and wild cherry bark or infuse it in raw honey to swallow by the spoonful.

Field garlic is most effective when consumed in large quantities. You want to be reeking of garlic, have it seeping from your pores—that's when you know you are using enough to help your lungs.

The leaves of field garlic are particularly useful for early spring colds and stuck congestion when used in combination with pine needles. Use this aromatic pairing in a delicious tea, sweetened with honey, to help loosen stuck mucus and open sinuses.

Future Harvests

Although field garlic is easy to find, and some consider it a troublesome weed, be a mindful harvester if you want to have access to field garlic each spring. By removing the bulb, you are removing the entire plant from the soil. Clipping the edible tops is the more sustainable way to enjoy this medicinal plant and ensure a steady supply each year.

HERBAL PREPARATIONS

Field garlic tea
Infusion
Drink ¼ cup, 3 times per day.

ghost pipe

Monotropa uniflora
corpse plant, ghost plant, Indian pipe
PARTS USED aerial parts

Ghost pipe is a useful first aid remedy that helps ease pain caused by trauma, tension, migraines, or pinched nerves.

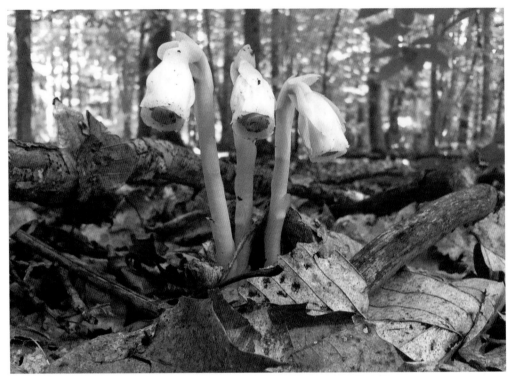

Ghost pipe is a bright, translucent white plant that lacks chlorophyll, which gives it an otherworldly appearance. It can be used acutely for pain caused by trauma in lieu of conventional pain relief medications.

How to Identify

Ghost pipe is a small, white, parasitic perennial. It is non-photosynthetic and contains no chlorophyll or green parts. Because of its ghostly white appearance, the plant is sometimes mistaken for a fungus. White, waxy, fleshy stems grow 4–12 inches tall, with smooth and white, scalelike leaves that alternate up the stem. Each stem holds a single bell-shaped white flower with 3–8 petals and 12 stamens; it blooms from early summer through early autumn, often after a few days of rainfall. As it produces seeds, the plant turns dark brown and black and dies.

Where, When, and How to Wildcraft

Ghost pipe grows in colonies in dense, moist forest understories with an abundance of surface leaf litter. The plant is not photosynthetic and depends on relationships with dead or decaying trees and associated mycorrhiza, especially species of *Russula* or *Lactarius*, for nutrients. When it is found, it is often growing near beech, maple, oak, or pine trees.

Wildcraft the bright white plant in the summer while it is in flower. Carefully clip off the tender tops and avoid disturbing the root system.

Medicinal Uses

Ghost pipe is a useful first aid remedy for easing pain caused by trauma in lieu of conventional pain relief medications. It also helps relieve skeletal tension associated with migraines and neck pain, as well as sharp, shooting pains associated with pinched nerves.

Use grain alcohol to make a tincture from ghost pipe. The plant material will turn a deep and gorgeous purple, with a subtle flavor reminiscent of bubblegum.

Future Harvests

Ghost pipe is a perennial plant, but it is not abundant in all woodland areas. Wildcraft only the aerial parts according to the abundance of plants in the area. Be careful not to disturb the roots.

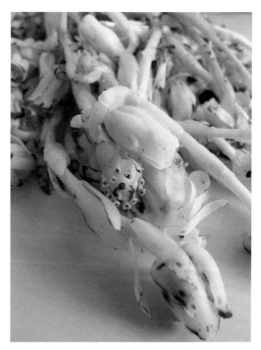

Ghost pipe grows in small colonies. Take care not to remove the underground root system when harvesting. Wildcraft the plant while it is in flower and is bright white, clipping only the tops.

HERBAL PREPARATIONS

Ghost pipe tincture
1 part fresh flowers and stems, chopped
2 parts menstruum (50 percent alcohol, 50 percent distilled water)
Take 7–10 drops as needed.

ginkgo

Ginkgo biloba
PARTS USED fruit, leaves

While ginkgo nuts and leaves are traditional plant medicines used throughout Asia, the leaves are also popular in Western plant-based medicine, commonly used in teas available in health food stores. Ginkgo supports overall brain health and increases clarity and mental function.

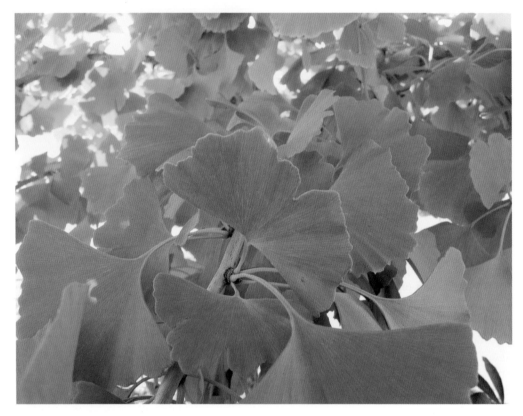

Ginkgo leaves are uniquely shaped and textured, which makes the tree easy to identify. Ginkgo is used to support overall brain health and to increase clarity and mental function.

How to Identify

Ginkgo trees in the wild can reach up to 100 feet tall, but it is more common to find the tree growing from 30 to 60 feet tall, particularly when it is planted as a landscape ornamental.

As the tree ages, its gray bark becomes cracked and deeply furrowed. The fan-shaped leaves are handsomely double-lobed and deeply veined, bright green in the summer and turning to golden yellow hues in the fall.

Most ginkgo trees in the landscape are male plants, because female trees produce a small, putrid-smelling, peach-colored fruit in the fall that makes a mess when it drops on city sidewalks and trails. The fruit, however, contains a nutritious and edible nut that is delicious. The odor of the female ginkgo fruit is unmistakable: sharp and ripe, and reminiscent of rotting cheese—or a good smelly cheese, depending on your taste.

Where, When, and How to Wildcraft

The ginkgo tree prefers rich, well-drained soil, but it is tolerant of drought conditions and thrives in a variety of growing conditions, including polluted urban environments. Its unusual leaves make it fairly easy to spot. Leaves are ready to harvest when they turn golden yellow in late fall, about the time of the first frost.

Wildcraft leaves from trees that are not growing in a main thoroughfare or in heavily trafficked urban areas to avoid leaves contaminated with auto emissions and other city pollutants. To collect them, place a sheet beneath the tree or branch and shake the tree. Dry the leaves on a screen or in a food dehydrator for use in tea.

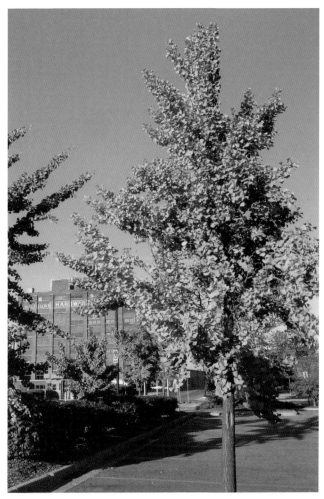

Ginkgo is an ancient native tree that was once distributed widely across Asia and North America. It is commonly grown in North America as a landscape ornamental.

Medicinal Uses

Prepare the dry yellow leaves for tea; boiling the leaves extracts the most minerals for the brew. As a functional food, ginkgo fruit can be added to your diet to promote brain health. It offers a mineral cocktail of copper, niacin, phosphorus, potassium, and thiamine. Once shelled, the nutmeats can be roasted, toasted, or boiled to improve and maximize their digestibility.

Future Harvests

Ginkgo is a common ornamental tree across the Midwest, and you can wildcraft the

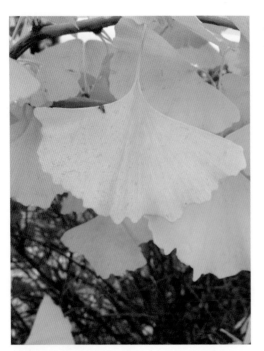

Gather bright yellow ginkgo leaves in the fall for tea. Boiling the leaves extracts the most minerals for the brew.

fruits and falling leaves without affecting future harvests.

Cautions, Concerns, and Considerations

Wear gloves when you wildcraft and work with ginkgo fruit. Compounds in the ripe fruit can irritate sensitive skin and cause a rash.

HERBAL PREPARATIONS

Ginkgo leaf tea
Decoction
Drink 1 cup per day.

---

goldenrod

Solidago species
PARTS USED flowers, leaves

*Goldenrod is a valuable wild medicine for use as a diuretic for the urinary
tract and a lymphatic herb to support musculoskeletal issues such as bursitis.*

How to Identify

More than 20 species of goldenrod are distributed across the Midwest, and all possess similar properties and can be used interchangeably.

Goldenrod's clumping perennial stalks grow to 5 feet tall. Oblong, lance-shaped leaves begin in a basal rosette, and silver-green, hairy leaves alternate up the stalk. The plant blooms as early as mid-August, with small, hairy, yellow flowers arranged in dense sprays that hang heavy in the summer sun.

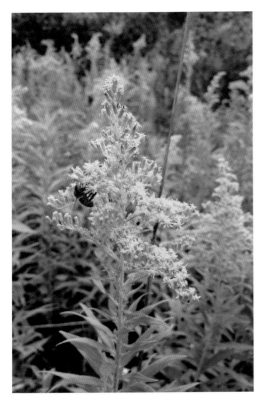

Follow the honey bees to wildcraft goldenrod.
They will be busy beneath the sunshine, gathering
nectar and pollen.

Where, When, and How to Wildcraft

Goldenrod thrives in prairies and open fields and along roads and riverbanks in full sun. Honey bees are usually busy working in the goldenrod flowers, gathering nectar and pollen, and their activity signifies an opportune time to wildcraft the plant. Use your senses of taste and smell to determine which plants are most aromatic.

Wildcraft the entire stalks with leaves and flowers throughout the summer and fall when the weather is warm, dry, and sunny. Do not harvest the plant on a wet and rainy day, because it will be less aromatic in damp weather.

Drying the tiny flowers can be a challenge, because they go to seed almost immediately and make a frustrating mess. Dry the plant by hanging bundles inside a loose-fitting paper bag to catch the flowers and seeds as they fall.

Medicinal Uses

Goldenrod is a valuable wild plant to add to the herbalist's apothecary. Its flavors are aromatic and predominantly bitter. The plant is also astringent, making the tongue feel dry upon tasting the leaves or drinking the tea.

Prepared as a hot tea, dry or fresh goldenrod will be predominantly bitter, sending a shudder up and down your spine; it's also astringent, with that dry-up-your-mouth sensation.

Chewing goldenrod flowers or a leaf or two in the field has a carminative effect that can help with an upset stomach. A tea made of leaves and flowers can help as well. A strong hot brew is quite bitter, so steep the plant for only a few minutes. Then cover and strain the tea to catch any of the hairs from the plant, which can cause irritation.

Contrary to popular belief, goldenrod is not the cause of hay fever in the summer. Instead, ragweed (*Ambrosia* species) should be blamed for that, with its microscopic windborne pollen. Goldenrod pollen is too heavy to be airborne and thus is not the source of late summer allergies.

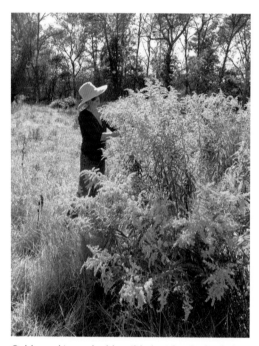

Goldenrod is a valuable wild plant for the herbalist's apothecary. It can be used as an aromatic bitter, a diuretic for the urinary tract, and a lymphatic to support musculoskeletal injuries like bursitis.

In fact, goldenrod is the hay fever allergy antidote. Its astringent qualities can effectively dry up leaky, drippy eyes and noses, and it helps soothe postnasal drip that results not only from summer and spring allergies, but also from animal dander allergies. Combine goldenrod with ground ivy, New England aster, and nettle in tea to create an excellent allergy reliever.

Herbalists also use goldenrod as a diuretic. The tea is helpful to astringe urinary tissues during a urinary tract infection. The plant is also valuable prepared as a liniment compress (using tea or an extract) or extracted in olive oil to make a salve for arthritis, sore muscles, or soft-tissue complaints. It blends well with mullein, St. John's wort, and yarrow for these uses.

Future Harvests

Goldenrod is an abundant wildflower throughout the Midwest, and wildcrafting a few bundles of flowers in the summer sun will not harm the plant's future sustainability.

HERBAL PREPARATIONS

Goldenrod tea
Infusion
Drink 1 cup as needed, or use externally for a compress.

Goldenrod tincture
1 part fresh flowers and leaves, chopped
2 parts menstruum (50 percent alcohol, 50 percent distilled water)
Take 10–15 drops as needed.

Goldenrod-infused oil
1 part fresh flowers and leaves, chopped
2 parts oil
Use for massage.

grindelia

Grindelia squarrosa
curlycup gumweed
PARTS USED flowers, leaves

Grindelia's resinous blossoms and leaves are effective for relieving and relaxing the muscle tension resulting from a wet, whooping, or barking cough.

How to Identify
Grindelia is a coarse biennial or perennial herb, 12–24 inches tall, with branching green stems. Its blossoms and leaves are excessively sticky with resin. Leaves are arranged alternately and are small and oblong with wavy margins, and they are often dotted with resinous glands. Each leaf has a tiny hard tooth at its tip. In midsummer, backward-curling, scaly bracts surround the bright yellow rays of petals, with 14–16 petals circling a yellow center.

Where, When, and How to Wildcraft
Look for grindelia in the sandy dune regions or sandy upper elevations of the Midwest, and along disturbed roadsides and streamsides throughout the region. Grindelia blooms in July and August. Wildcraft the flower buds, blossoms, and leaves when the plant is in full bloom.

Medicinal Uses
The resinous grindelia is helpful to relax a wet, whooping, barking cough. It will ease the spasmodic heaving and can be blended with other plants such as elecampane to increase expectoration.

Prepare fresh grindelia as a tincture in a high-proof alcohol to extract the resins. Blend it with goldenrod, mullein, New England aster, and copious amounts of garlic to dry up damp and wet bacterial infections.

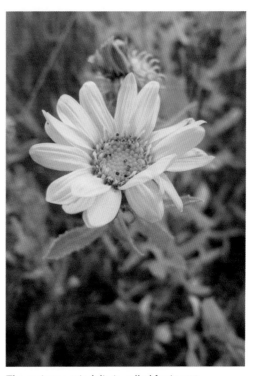

The resinous grindelia is called for in wet, whooping, barking dry coughs. As a relaxant it will ease the spasmodic heaving, and blended with other plants like elecampane it can increase expectoration.

Because of its resinous, sticky nature, grindelia is less effective as a water-based preparation such as tea. To temper grindelia's drying nature, consider adding honey to soothe tense and constricted tissues.

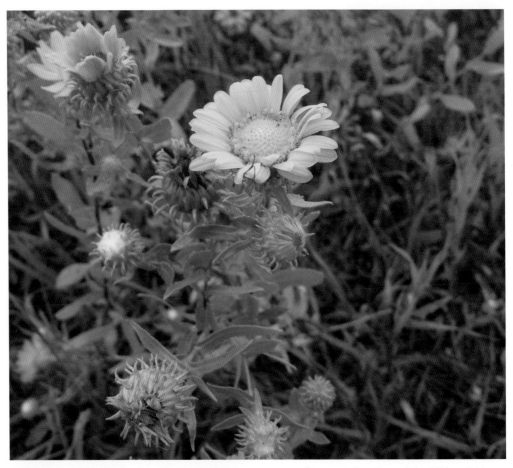

Wildcraft grindelia flowers from the sandy dune regions or sandy upper elevations of the Midwest. Harvest the blossoms in high summer of July and August when the plants are in full bloom.

Future Harvests

Although grindelia can be invasive in some areas, it is an important plant for medicinal uses and pollinators such as bees. Harvest the buds and flowers in limited amounts and help cultivate new wild stands of the plants with cuttings.

HERBAL PREPARATIONS

Grindelia tea
Decoction
Drink ¼ cup as needed.

Grindelia tincture
1 part fresh flowers and leaves, chopped
2 parts menstruum (95 percent alcohol, 5 percent distilled water)
Take 10 drops as needed.

ground ivy

Glechoma hederacea
creeping Charlie, gill-over-the-ground
PARTS USED flowers, leaves, stems

Although some homeowners declare ground ivy to be the enemy of a perfect lawn, it is a useful herbal remedy. This aromatic and astringent plant is helpful in alleviating head and chest congestion and can dry up leaky and drippy sinuses.

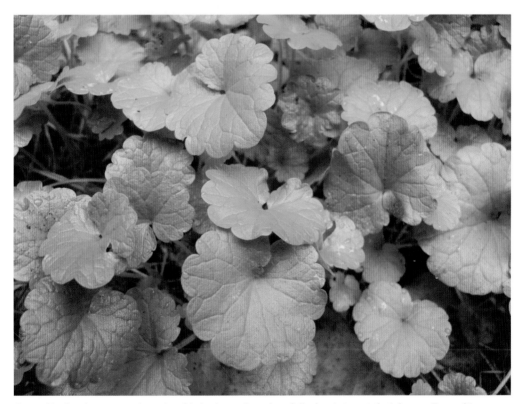

Ground ivy's minty aroma is noticeable in the spring when folks begin to cut their lawns. Ground ivy can alleviate head and chest congestion, and dries up drippy sinuses caused by allergies.

How to Identify

Ground ivy is a small and creeping mint that grows to about 6 inches tall. It spreads by runners. Small, soft, heart-shaped leaves are arranged oppositely on square stems. Small purple flowers bloom in late May, and the entire plant emits a fragrant minty scent when crushed.

Where, When, and How to Wildcraft

Interspersed with dandelions, dock, and grass, ground ivy sometimes grows thick like a carpet. In mid- to late spring, harvest ground ivy easily by hand or using kitchen shears, but be careful not to include any nearby grasses or you will be picking out those blades in the kitchen. After ground ivy blooms, it begins to die back a bit and turns dry and rough like many other mints.

Wildcraft ground ivy as cleanly as possible, because it is difficult to remove embedded dust and debris from the small hairs on the plant, even with washing. Washing will rinse out the aromatics of the plant as well.

Medicinal Uses

Use ground ivy fresh; the aromatic properties are significantly lost upon drying or dehydrating. Other mints such as spotted bee balm and wild bergamot are better choices if you want to dry an aromatic mint-family plant for tea.

Ground ivy is helpful in alleviating head and chest congestion. Prepare flowers, leaves, and stems as a hot tea, covering the tea while steeping to preserve the aromatic compounds. It also makes a great chest-clearing steam inhalation.

For a combination to dry up leaky, drippy sinus congestion caused by hay fever, environmental allergies, or animal allergies, mix ground ivy tincture with equal parts goldenrod, nettle, and New England aster tinctures to stop the runny nose in its tracks.

Future Harvests

Ground ivy is frequently considered a persistent nuisance by homeowners who want a perfectly groomed landscape. Wildcrafting the plant poses little threat to this dandy and abundant little weed.

Cautions, Concerns, and Considerations

Ground ivy takes up minerals into its stem and leaves, so be sure to wildcraft in an area where you are familiar with the soil quality to avoid potentially contaminated plants.

HERBAL PREPARATIONS

Ground ivy tea
Infusion
Drink ¼ cup as needed.

Ground ivy tincture
1 part fresh flowers, leaves, and stems, chopped
2 parts menstruum (50 percent alcohol, 50 percent distilled water)
Take 10 drops as needed.

---

hawkweed

Hieracium species
PARTS USED aerial parts

Hawkweed is useful in alleviating head and chest congestion and works similarly as a bronchodilator in asthma that has been triggered by environmental particulates.

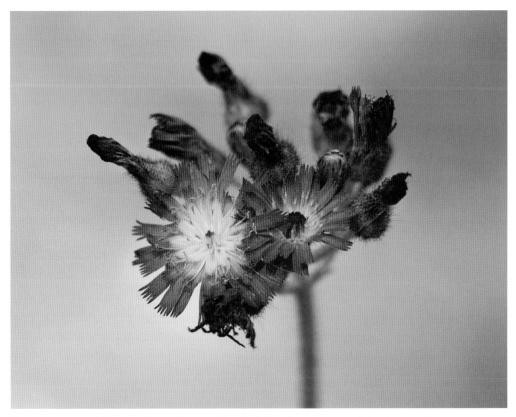

Orange hawkweed (*H. aurantiacum*) is useful in alleviating damp sinus and chest congestion.

How to Identify

Hawkweed is a small perennial with a basal rosette that produces several erect and fibrous stalks, 10–36 inches tall. Clusters of orange-red (*H. aurantiacum*) or yellow (*H. caespitosum*) rays of flowers bloom from late June to early July. Both flowers and leaves exude a sticky white sap when cut or broken.

Where, When, and How to Wildcraft

Find hawkweed in disturbed sites or along the edges of woodlands, where it grows in partial shade to full sun. Look for the colorful blooms in early to midsummer. Wildcraft the aerial parts of the plant and prepare fresh or dry for later use.

Medicinal Uses

Sticky and resinous, hawkweed is useful in alleviating damp sinus and chest congestion. It works similarly to New England aster by relaxing the bronchial tubes and lungs in asthma triggered by environmental particulates. Because it is resinous, hawkweed is best prepared as a tincture extract in high-proof alcohol, but it can also be prepared as a hot tea. Cover the tea while steeping to preserve the aroma.

For wet and damp lung conditions, hawkweed works well with aromatic plants such as butterfly weed, elecampane, and grindelia. Consider adding garlic if infection is involved. For a combination to alleviate leaky, drippy sinus congestion caused by hay fever, environmental allergies, or animal allergies, mix hawkweed with equal parts goldenrod, ground ivy, nettle, and New England aster to stop the runny nose in its tracks.

Future Harvests

Hawkweed is deemed invasive in some areas and is sparsely distributed in other areas across the Midwest. Harvest aerial parts according to abundance.

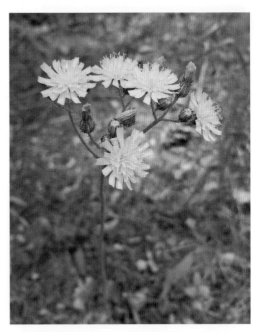

Yellow hawkweed (*H. caespitosum*) is used similarly to orange hawkweed, though it can be a bit less resinous.

HERBAL PREPARATIONS

Hawkweed tea
Decoction
Drink ¼ cup as needed.

Hawkweed tincture
1 part fresh flowers, leaves, and stems, chopped
2 parts menstruum (95 percent alcohol, 5 percent distilled water)
Take 10 drops as needed.

hawthorn

Crataegus species
haw, thornapple
PARTS USED flowers, fruit, leaves, thorns

A tree full of lore, hawthorn has a long history of use and scientific research as a heart medicine and tonic. It is a valuable remedy for strengthening and tonifying the heart.

How to Identify
Hawthorn is a deciduous shrub or tree that can reach 30 feet in height at maturity. The tree bark is dark brown and scaly. Unbranched thorns 1½ to 3 inches long grow along the dense branches. Whitish five-petaled flowers bloom in mid-May. Technically a pome, or tiny apple, the red

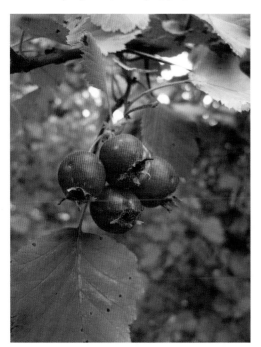

Hawthorn has a long history as a heart medicine and tonic. It is frequently used in herbal protocols to support tonifying the heart muscle and vascular system.

fruit is about 1 inch in diameter and hangs in clusters that ripen in early September.

Where, When, and How to Wildcraft
You'll find hawthorn growing in fields and hedgerows. Once you are familiar with the tree's shape, you will be able to see it from afar, with its dense, seemingly windblown form.

Hawthorn branches are spiked with long thorns, warning wildcrafters to hone their senses and pay attention, lest they fall into the shrub's spiny clutches while wildcrafting the leaves, pretty blossoms, or delicious fruits.

Wildcraft the flowers, leaves, and thorns in midspring, around Mother's Day. Be sure to leave some blossoms on the tree for pollination; they will ripen into tiny pomes ready for harvest by early September. When the fruit ripens, place a sheet under the tree and gently shake its branches to release the fruit from higher branches.

Medicinal Uses
Hawthorn is frequently used in herbal protocols to tonify the heart muscle and vascular system that has been damaged or is under stress from excess inflammation. High cholesterol, a signifier of excess inflammation, and high blood pressure are indicators for hawthorn. It is used in more complex herbal

A Magical Hawthorn Harvest

An abundance of literature covers the use of hawthorn berries, flowers, leaves, and thorns for support of the heart. But I like to focus on the hawthorn's effect on me and my internal rhythm.

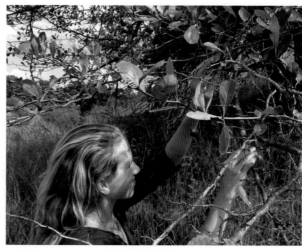

Wildcrafting the berries and thorns.

One fair September day, I was called out to the fields in search of my hawthorn tree—a tree of the faeries, a tree that in folklore is linked with the spiritual heart, fertility, and death.

Approaching this tree in a windy field, I felt overcome with calm. The winds, swirling about me and within me, calmed. The hawthorn's branches, spiked with 3-inch thorns, warned me to hone my senses and pay attention to the placement of my person, lest I lose an eye. I took each step carefully as I came close; I was on a rocky hillside and it wasn't in my interest to fall into her spiny clutches.

As I sat in the soft grass at the base of the tree, a profound and deep sense of peace came over me. I collected the newly fallen fruits and felt my senses sharpen, as my ability to focus my attention increased. Colors became more vibrant. Even today, those colors are burned into my memory. The wisdom offered to me that day was to quiet down and find peace and softness.

The cooling nature of hawthorn berries helps bring a sense of peace to anyone who is feeling agitated. Good for a person who has a limited ability to settle down and pay attention, they can help bring the attention inward.

Hawthorn can soften the ache of broken-heartedness. And for anyone who has a hard time being playful, hawthorn can help bring a bit of softness to a hardened heart. It teaches us how to be open and willing to receive soft, loving, nourishing kindness in a way that is respectful of space and boundaries.

I like to prepare the berries, which I harvest at peak ripeness, with dried leaves and flowers I've gathered earlier in the spring into a brandy-based elixir, sweetened with raw honey. It's divine to take a drop here and there whenever I feel an achy, melancholic anxiety in my spiritual heart. It offers a peaceful calm.

protocols in severe conditions, frequently as a tincture of the thorn, and is usually recommended alongside a diet rich in healthy fats and low in omega 6 and refined sugars to help restore the body's lipids and circulatory and vascular systems.

As a functional food, hawthorn fruit is high in flavonoids and antioxidants, which are naturally good for the heart and can help reduce inflammation. Use the fruit similarly to crabapple for cooking and making hard cider.

Many herbalists have a special place in their hearts for the magic of the hawthorn. With a rich history in folklore, hawthorn fruits and flowers can be made into tinctures and used energetically to ease the heart of sadness and grief. An elixir of honey and brandy makes an especially nice energetic heart elixir. The thorns can be tinctured with the fruit to use as a talisman for protection or to help support someone who wants to maintain proper boundaries in daily life, but may have trouble saying no.

Future Harvests

The hawthorn reproduces easily; birds are a big help, because they love the fruit and spread its seeds. Mindfully wildcraft fallen fruit to avoid impacting future harvests.

Cautions, Concerns, and Considerations

Many hawthorns suffer from rust blight that affects other plants in the Rosaceae family. This affects both the leaves and fruits, causing them to fall from the tree as early as August. The blighted fruits are edible, but they are blemished and often not as juicy or ripe as the fruit that are unaffected and remain on the tree until they are ripe.

Because hawthorn is known to be a plant of the faery realm, it's always worth remembering to take a gift of butter for the plant faeries and to sing songs while harvesting the fruit and thorns. At the very least—and if you don't believe in the plant faeries— singing songs or whistling is a good way to express thanks and gratitude for the tree's fruits as you harvest them.

HERBAL PREPARATIONS

Hawthorn tincture
1 part fresh or dry flowers, fruit, leaves, and thorns, chopped
2 parts menstruum (95 percent alcohol, 5 percent distilled water)
Take 10–15 drops as needed.

honeysuckle

Lonicera japonica
PARTS USED flowers

As a plant medicine, honeysuckle blossom is a valuable herb to use at the onset of a cold or flu. It also makes a delightful honey infusion and refreshing iced tea.

How to Identify

Honeysuckle is a vining plant with oppositely arranged, oblong, glossy leaves that can sometimes remain on the plant throughout winter, though it is not always evergreen in colder climates.

Tubular white flowers form in pairs along the stem. They are sweetly aromatic but taste predominantly bitter. The nectar inside the base of the flower, however, is sweet and tasty. The flowers fade to light yellow as they age. Honeysuckle berries are black and inedible.

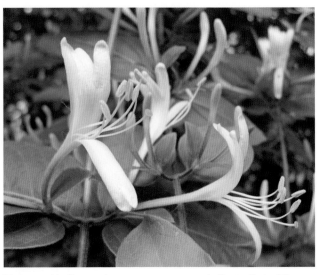

Honeysuckle flowers have a sweet aroma similar to that of the intoxicating jasmine or orange blossom.

Where, When, and How to Wildcraft

This rambling vine loves to climb. Honeysuckle grows wild over fences, shrubs, and fallen trees at the edges and interiors of woodlands. You'll find it growing in stream valleys, as well as in hot, dry waste places, though it tolerates shade.

Look for the heavily fragrant blossoms in mid-June as the temperatures begin to warm and their scent hangs heavy on the breeze. Pick the flowers by hand; they will quickly wilt. Preserve them in honey, make a tincture, or dry them for tea and store them in an airtight container to preserve the sweet aromatics.

Medicinal Uses

Honeysuckle blossom is aromatic and bitter and can be used as a diaphoretic to help the body produce sweat. It is a useful herb at the onset of a cold or flu, particularly with chills or excess heat as the body begins to initiate a fever to ward off a virus. Use honeysuckle in place of elderflower as a relaxant febrifuge, or fever-reducer. It also combines well with boneset, mints such as wild bergamot and spotted bee balm, and yarrow.

Captured as a culinary herb, honeysuckle makes a wonderful iced tea. A cool infusion of honeysuckle, combined with lemon balm and rose petals and garnished with fresh mint, makes a refreshing and aromatic beverage.

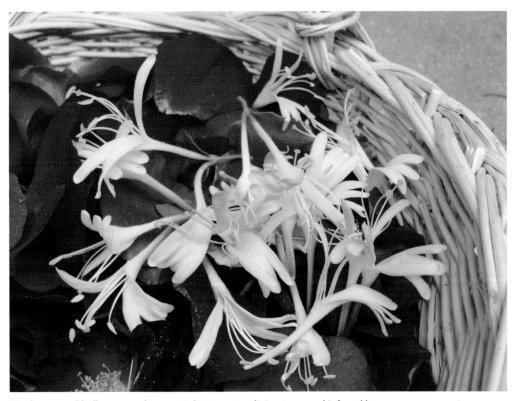

Use honeysuckle flowers and rose petals to create elixirs, teas, and infused honeys.

To preserve the seductive flower's enticing aroma, infuse fresh blossoms in raw honey. Add fresh, unwilted blossoms to a jar, and cover them with raw honey. Let the mixture infuse for at least several weeks, occasionally turning the jar upside down to stir up the plant material. Strain the honey for use.

Future Harvests

Honeysuckle is an invasive plant, and wild-crafting the flowers will not significantly affect its future growth.

HERBAL PREPARATIONS

Honeysuckle tea
Infusion
Drink ¼ cup as needed.

Honeysuckle tincture
1 part fresh flowers
2 parts menstruum (50 percent alcohol, 50 percent distilled water)
Take 10–15 drops as needed.

Honeysuckle-infused honey
1 part fresh flowers, chopped
3 parts raw, unpasteurized honey
Use as needed.

horehound

Marrubium species
PARTS USED flowers, leaves, stems

Horehound is an age-old remedy for colds, hacking coughs, and stuck lung congestion. Wildcraft the plant to make soothing cough drops, syrups, and herbal pastilles.

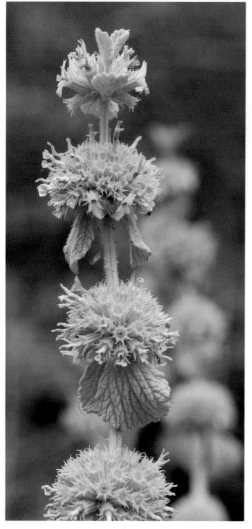

Horehound flowers form in clusters along the stem. Horehound is a classic remedy for colds and stuck lung congestion.

How to Identify

Horehound is a clumping perennial in the mint family that grows to 3 feet tall. Its stems are square, woody, and branching, with alternately arranged, small and hairy, gray-green, wrinkled, heart-shaped leaves. Clusters of small white flowers grow in whorls along the stem at the terminal axes of the leaves. The entire plant is aromatic and slightly bitter in flavor.

Where, When, and How to Wildcraft

Look for horehound in poor soils. It tolerates partial to full sun. Wildcraft the leaves, stems, and flowers while the plant is in bloom in the summer. Use horehound fresh in tinctures, teas, or syrups, or dry it for later use.

Medicinal Uses

Grind the dry herb into a powder and prepare it as a useful and soothing throat drop made with honey, or combine it with equal parts powdered licorice roots, marshmallow roots, rose petals, and slippery elm bark. Use the throat drops to soothe a dry, scratchy throat and facilitate expectoration of stuck mucus in the lungs.

Horehound can also be infused in honey with herbs such as cherry bark, licorice root, marshmallow root, mullein leaf, and slippery elm to soothe and calm spasmodic coughing and facilitate more productive expectoration.

A hot tea of horehound, combined with elder-flower, spotted bee balm, or wild bergamot, is a relaxant to offer during a cold or flu.

Future Harvests

Horehound is a perennial mint that reproduces easily with cuttings or by seed. Harvesting aerial parts will not significantly affect its future growth or harvests.

HERBAL PREPARATIONS

Horehound tea
Infusion
Drink ½ cup as needed.

Horehound tincture
1 part fresh flowers, leaves, and stems, chopped
2 parts menstruum (95 percent alcohol, 5 percent distilled water)
Take 10–15 drops as needed.

Horehound-infused honey
1 part fresh flowers and leaves, chopped
3 parts raw, unpasteurized honey
Use as needed.

horsetail

Equisetum species
mare's tail, snakegrass
PARTS USED aerial parts

*For those who have bone density or arthritis issues or connective tissue injuries,
or for those who want to rely less on synthetic sources of mineral supplements,
horsetail is a plant to integrate into the apothecary.*

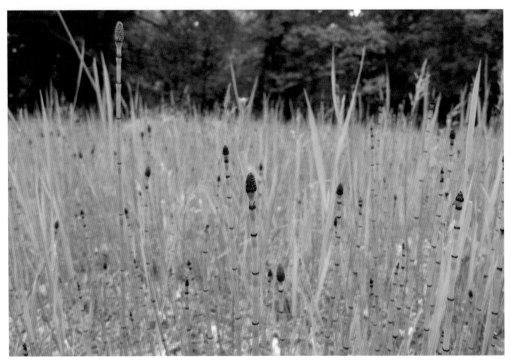

Horsetail is high in minerals, specifically silica, which is foundational in maintaining healthy skin, hair, and nails. Boiling fresh or dried horsetail to create a broth will extract the silica as well as the other minerals in the plant.

How to Identify

Horsetail is a perennial plant with erect stems that reach 3–4 feet tall. The leaves are arranged in whorls, fused together to wrap around the stem in nodal sheaths. Horsetail stems are unique; they are jointed, dry to the touch, coarse, and hollow, and they are either fertile or sterile.

Fertile stems grow in the spring, are low-growing, and range in color from brown to white. Sterile stems are green; they grow taller and produce whorls of fine, feathery branches. Both stem types are topped by a dark strobile, a cone-shaped mass of spore-bearing scales.

Where, When, and How to Wildcraft

Look for horsetail growing along the banks of streams and rivers, in wetlands, and in dunes. You can harvest the aerial parts from mid- to late spring and into the fall, but traditionally the green sterile stems are wildcrafted in the spring before the feathery branches unfurl in summer.

Clip the upper parts of the stems with substantial kitchen shears or pruners, and then cut the stems down to smaller sizes and dry them completely for storage in an airtight container. As far as quality goes, like nearly all wildcrafted plants, wildcrafted horsetail is leaps and bounds better in quality than the dried horsetail available commercially.

Medicinal Uses

Horsetail is an ancient plant that is high in minerals, specifically silica, which is foundational in maintaining healthy skin, hair, and nails. Boil fresh or dried horsetail to create a broth that extracts the silica and other minerals in the plant. Drink it as is or use it in cooking to add minerals to other foods, especially starches and grains.

Use the delicious, mineral-rich broth as a hot or iced tea, or use it as a vegan broth for soups, stews, and smoothies. Horsetail's flavor is neutral, and it works well in combination with many other herbs. Add horsetail directly to a simmering pot of bone broth, and then strain it off with other ingredients before consuming the broth. Combine it with other mineral-dense herbs such as bull kelp (a large seaweed), nettle, oatstraw, and red clover.

Future Harvests

Clip the aerial parts of the plant and leave its root system in place to ensure the plant's sustainability. Horsetail grows abundantly in wetlands and dune areas, but habitat loss has impacted its distribution.

Cautions, Concerns, and Considerations

Wildcraft the plants in locales that are free from heavy metal pollution; lead and other harmful minerals can be taken up by the plant.

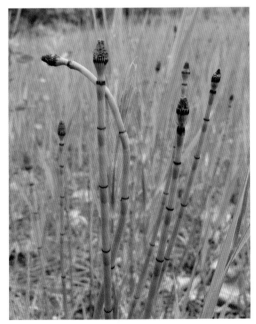

Wildcraft the aerial parts of horsetail throughout the year.

HERBAL PREPARATIONS

Horsetail tea
Decoction
Drink 1 cup per day.

Horsetail tincture
1 part fresh aerial parts, chopped
2 parts menstruum (95 percent alcohol,
   5 percent distilled water)
Take 10 drops as needed.

hyssop

Agastache scrophulariifolia
purple giant hyssop
PARTS USED flowers, leaves, stems

Hyssop is a classic remedy for colds, hacking coughs, and stuck lung congestion.
Use it to make soothing cough drops, cough syrups, and herbal pastilles.

How to Identify
Hyssop is a clumping perennial plant in the mint family.
It grows to 6 feet in height,
with ovate and pointed leaves
arranged oppositely on square
stems. Flowers in the dense,
pink-to-purple flower spike
begin blooming in mid- to late
summer and do not all bloom
simultaneously.

Where, When, and How to Wildcraft
Hyssop prefers damp soil, and
you'll find it growing along
the edges of woodlands and
in riparian areas adjacent to
wetlands or streams. It grows
in areas with partial sun, often
alongside other native wildflowers such as spotted bee
balm and yarrow.

   Collect flowers throughout
the summer and take a stem
here and there from each plant,
being careful not to disturb
the bees collecting nectar and
pollen from the flowers. Bundle
the stems to dry, or use them fresh. Store
the dried stems and leaves in an airtight
container to preserve the hyssop's aromatic
compounds.

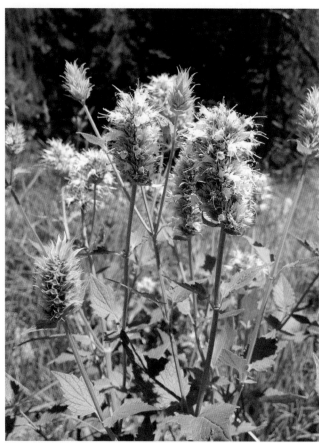

Wild hyssop, with its showy purple flower spike of midsummer, is
an aromatic herb that you can dry for a winter tea, or you can use
its leaves as a tincture or to infuse honey.

Medicinal Uses
Dry this aromatic herb to use in a winter tea,
or use its leaves in a tincture or infused in
honey. Dry hyssop can be ground and mixed

with honey as a useful and soothing throat drop, or combine it with equal parts powdered licorice root, marshmallow root, rose petal, sage, and slippery elm. These pastilles can help soothe a dry, scratchy throat and facilitate expectoration of stuck mucus in the lungs.

Hyssop can also be prepared as a honey infusion along with herbs such as cherry bark, licorice root, marshmallow root, mullein leaf, and slippery elm to soothe and calm spasmodic coughing and facilitate more productive expectoration. Or create a tasty hyssop and maple syrup blend.

Future Harvests

Wild hyssop is not rare, but it isn't as prolific across the Midwest as it once was. Habitat loss has affected this plant, and you can assist with its future sustainability by helping propagate the plant with cuttings. The honey bees will appreciate your effort.

HERBAL PREPARATIONS

Hyssop tea
Infusion
Drink ½ cup as needed.

Hyssop syrup
1 part hyssop tea infusion
1 part maple syrup
Use as needed.

Hyssop tincture
1 part fresh flowers, leaves, and stems, chopped
2 parts menstruum (50 percent alcohol, 50 percent distilled water)
Take 10–15 drops as needed.

Hyssop-infused honey
1 part fresh flowers and leaves, chopped
3 parts raw, unpasteurized honey
Use as needed.

jewelweed

Impatiens capensis
touch-me-not
PARTS USED flowers, leaves, stems

Jewelweed is a familiar plant to all herbalists as a useful herbal remedy that helps astringe and soothe the itch caused by a poison ivy skin rash.

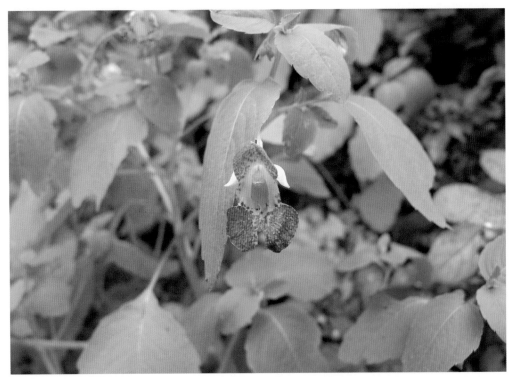

In July and August, jewelweed produces a beautiful tubular orange flower. It is a fast-growing plant that propagates by its abundant seed, easily released in the summer if anything brushes against the plant.

How to Identify

Jewelweed is a shallow-rooted, succulent annual that can grow in dense clumps like a ground cover. Water droplets that fall onto the leaves of the plant glisten like jewels because of the waxy leaf coating. This can make the entire plant shimmer, hence its common name.

The hollow stalks are a neon translucent green and 3–5 feet tall. Blue-green leaves are lanceolate with regular scalloped margins. The plant is very juicy when crushed. In July and August, jewelweed produces an inch-long, bilaterally symmetrical, trumpet-shaped orange flower, speckled in red. The fast-growing plant propagates by abundant seeds that are easily released in the summer when anything brushes against the plant.

Watch for Poison Ivy

Poison ivy (*Toxicodendron radicans*) is a common and unwelcome plant throughout the Midwest that grows in damp river valleys, woodlands and woodland edges, trailsides, sand dunes, and open fields. Although many have disdain for the plant, poison ivy offers helpful barriers to keep people away from land that may need time for healing or remediation, or land that has been heavily trafficked. It's nature's "No Trespassing" sign.

Notice where the plant grows before winter to avoid contacting the bare vines in the spring. "Leaves of three, let them be" may be a good start to identifying poison ivy, but the plant takes many shapes: a small and leafy creeping plant, a berry-producing vine in the fall, or a leafless, hairy vine in winter. Its compound leaves alternate along the woody stem. Poison ivy can be easily confused with young box elder trees, but box elder leaves grow in an opposite arrangement.

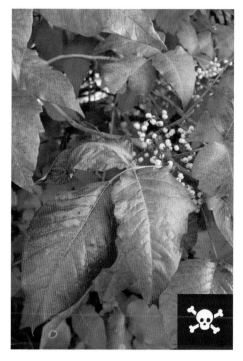 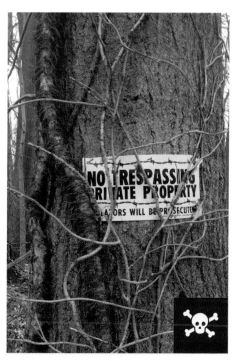

Tiny white poison ivy berries are produced in the fall, as leaves begin to turn.

The hairy vines of winter poison ivy are nature's "No Trespassing" sign.

Where, When, and How to Wildcraft

Look for jewelweed growing along the edges of streams, ditches, and woodlands. It often grows alongside poison ivy and nettle in the same moist habitat. Harvest stems and leaves in mid- to late summer, and pick the flowers in summer. The plant has a shallow root system that is easily removed from the soil.

Medicinal Uses

Jewelweed is most known for its effectiveness in helping counter the results of exposure to poison ivy and as a wash for the weepy rash the ivy can cause. For field use, crush the plant by hand for a makeshift poultice and apply it to the entire affected area. Apply the plant directly to the skin to help soothe the itch.

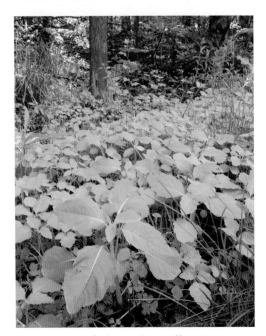

Jewelweed is most known for its effectiveness to help counter the results of exposure to poison ivy and as a wash for the weepy rash the poison ivy can cause. For field use, crush the plant by hand for a makeshift poultice and apply to the entire exposed area.

In the kitchen, heat jewelweed in water and strain it to use when cooled for a skin wash to soothe and astringe a poison ivy rash. Use other astringent plants in a wash in combination with jewelweed, such as apple bark, oak bark, and rose petals.

Jewelweed extracted into apple cider vinegar also makes an excellent astringent wash for the rash. Store jewelweed-infused vinegar in the refrigerator to use as needed throughout the season, or freeze the crushed plant into ice cube trays to use later. Soap-makers like to process jewelweed into poison ivy soap.

Future Harvests

Jewelweed spreads easily by seeds and grows quickly in large stands. Harvesting a few stalks for use in a medicinal remedy won't impact future harvests.

Cautions, Concerns, and Considerations

Jewelweed often grows alongside poison ivy and stinging nettle in the same moist habitat. Be careful to avoid contacting these plants when walking through the area to collect jewelweed.

HERBAL PREPARATIONS

Jewelweed topical wash
Decoction
Use topically as a skin wash or poultice.

Jewelweed-infused vinegar
1 part fresh flowers, leaves, and stems, chopped
2 parts vinegar
Use topically as an astringent skin wash, as needed.

Joe Pye weed

Eupatorium species
gravel root
PARTS USED aerial parts, roots

Herbalists use the roots of Joe Pye weed as a medicinal diuretic for urinary tract infections and kidney stones.

How to Identify

Joe Pye weed is an herbaceous perennial that reaches 5–7 feet tall. Dark green leaves are slightly fuzzy, serrated, and lance-shaped, and they grow in a whorled arrangement up the stem. Tiny, vanilla-scented flowers open in flat umbels of white, pinkish white, or mauve blooms in late July to early August.

Where, When, and How to Wildcraft

Look for Joe Pye weed growing in damp soils on wooded slopes, wet meadows and thickets, and stream margins. You can use the entire plant for medicine, including the roots. Harvest leaves and stems in the summer before the flower buds open; use them fresh or dry and store them for later use. Harvest the roots in the fall after the flowers have died. Dig the roots easily in areas of sandy, moist soils.

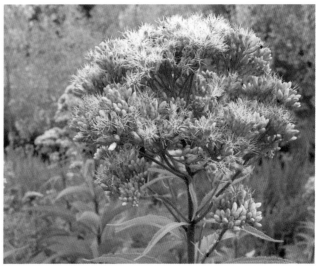

The flowers of Joe Pye weed open up in flat umbels of showy white or pinkish-white blooms in late July into early August.

Medicinal Use

Joe Pye weed is a useful herb to include in protocols to address urinary tract infections and kidney stones. Add other diuretic plants such as cranberry and goldenrod. When infection is present, echinacea is a helpful addition. With extreme spasmodic pain, add some wild yam.

For bursitis and damp joint conditions, use the plant's aerial parts as a poultice or use a tincture topically as a liniment. For back injury caused by swollen or ruptured discs, use Joe Pye weed with goldenseal and mullein root and leaf tinctures to help the body remove extra fluids, reabsorb the disc material, and heal the disc's ruptured membranes.

Future Harvests

Joe Pye weed is a perennial plant that may be regionally abundant, but because of the loss of wet meadow habitats, try to harvest the plant selectively and transplant plants from cuttings in your garden and in wild areas.

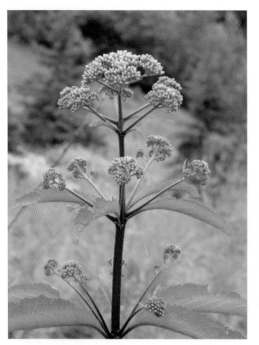

Clusters of tiny pink flower buds sprout from the tall stalks in summer.

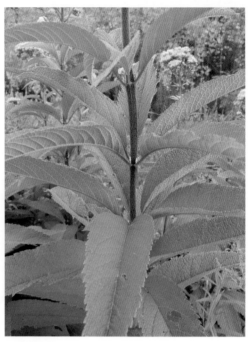

Joe Pye weed has slightly fuzzy, serrated, and pointed leaves that grow in a whorled arrangement up the stem.

Cautions, Concerns, and Considerations

Because Joe Pye weed readily grows in wet ditches, consider your harvesting location closely and avoid areas near industrial or factory farm run-off to avoid contamination.

HERBAL PREPARATIONS

Joe Pye weed tea
Decoction
Drink ½ cup per day.

Joe Pye weed tincture
1 part fresh flowers, leaves, and roots, chopped
2 parts menstruum (95 percent alcohol, 5 percent distilled water)
or
1 part dry flowers, leaves, and roots, chopped
4 parts menstruum (95 percent alcohol, 5 percent distilled water)
Take 10–15 drops as needed.

juniper

Juniperus communis

PARTS USED berries, leaves

Use astringent juniper leaves and berries as plant medicine to help clear sinuses and support kidney and urinary tract health.

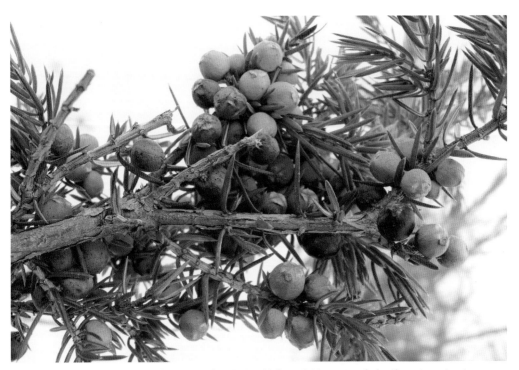

Juniper needle and berry tea is diuretic and antimicrobial, useful in protocols for the urinary tract system. The resinous aromatics of juniper can also be made into hot tea to open sinuses and ease upset digestion.

How to Identify

Juniper is a multistemmed coniferous shrub with dark reddish brown, shaggy bark. Low and spreading in exposed locations, it can reach 30 feet tall in some areas. Aromatic blue-green, needle-like leaves grow in whorls of three with a white band on the inner surface.

Juniper cones ripen in the fall as small, dusty blue, ¼ inch berrylike fruits that turn black when dry. Although the cones are not actual berries, they are commonly called berries.

Where, When, and How to Wildcraft

Juniper is widespread in areas of sandy, gravelly, or rocky, dry soil in fields and grasslands. It also grows on the dunes and shores of the Great Lakes and in ornamental garden plantings. Use shears to clip the leaves at any time; they are most aromatic in the spring.

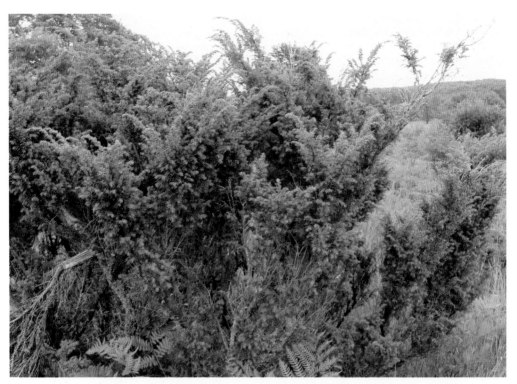

Stands of wild juniper grow in open spaces along the sandy dunes and shores of the Great Lakes.

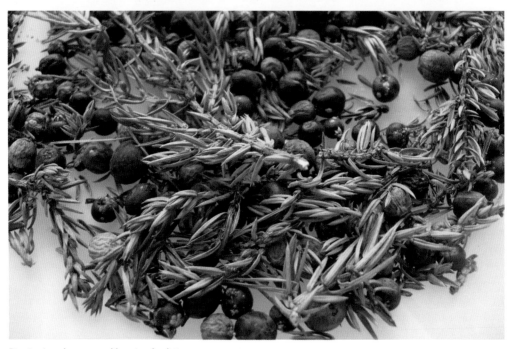

Dry juniper leaves and berries for later use.

Ripe berries can be easily collected by hand in late fall and winter. Dry the leaves and berries in a dehydrator, and then store them in airtight containers to preserve the aromatic compounds.

Medicinal Uses

A diuretic tea made with juniper leaves and berries is antimicrobial and useful in protocols to heal the urinary tract. As an astringent tea, it can be overly drying and should be blended accordingly with other herbs if used with goldenrod or Joe Pye weed. Blend it with cornsilk and cranberry to help heal urinary tract infections. Juniper is also used as part of kidney health protocols.

The tea is markedly astringent and is helpful in the field or kitchen to wash and dry up rashes such as those that arise from contact with poison ivy. Use the resinous aromatics of juniper in a sinus-clearing hot tea. Boil the leaves and berries in a covered pan for 20 minutes, remove it from the heat, and inhale the aromatic steam to clear the sinuses. Wildcraft berries and leaves for use in meat rubs and savory desserts, and for spicing cocktails.

Future Harvests

Juniper is abundant throughout the Midwest and can be propagated by cuttings.

HERBAL PREPARATIONS

Juniper tea
Decoction
Drink ¼ cup as needed, or use topically as a skin wash.

Juniper tincture
1 part fresh berries and leaves, chopped
2 parts menstruum (95 percent alcohol, 5 percent distilled water)
Take 10–15 drops as needed

---

lady's mantle

Alchemilla vulgaris
lion's foot
PARTS USED flowers, leaves, roots

*Showy lady's mantle is a beneficial astringent medicinal plant that is used
for wound care and as a tonic for both male and female reproductive systems.*

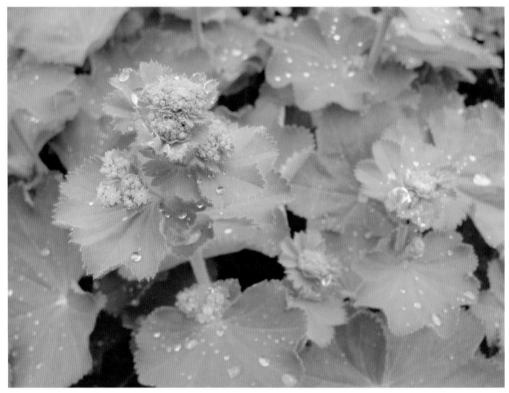

Lady's mantle perfectly catches morning dew droplets and raindrops after a storm, as they sparkle like diamonds on its leaves. Lady's mantle is an astringent herb used as a topical wash for wounds and to tone prolapsed tissues.

How to Identify

Lady's mantle is a small herbaceous perennial. Its kidney-shaped and finely toothed leaves, 3–5 inches in diameter, radiate from a common point on slender stalks up to 12 inches in length. Leaf undersides are silvery green. The entire plant is soft and slightly hairy.

The plant blooms in early to late summer, with terminal clusters of small yellow-green flowers. The entire plant lacks a significant aroma. The astringent rootstock is black, stout, and short.

Where, When, and How to Wildcraft

Look for lady's mantle in garden beds growing as a weed or growing in dappled shade among the violets and forget-me-nots. Wildcraft the flowers, leaves, and roots in the summer when the entire plant is in flower. Use the aerial parts fresh or dry them for later use. Lay the entire plant on a screen to dry; when dry, store them whole, crushing and preparing the plant at the time of use.

Medicinal Uses

The tannins in lady's mantle make it a particularly astringent plant. It's useful prepared as a topical wash for wound care. It is helpful in drying up wet and weepy rashes resulting from poison ivy and other irritants and septic infected wounds.

For these conditions, it mixes well with echinacea and plantain to clear or prevent septic infection. For wounds with bleeding, consider adding yarrow to help stanch the blood flow.

Traditionally, lady's mantle has been used as a female reproductive herb. It can be used in cases of uterine prolapse and is incorporated into protocols to strengthen vaginal tissues after birth. The plant combines well with raspberry leaves, red clover, and yarrow. Lady's mantle can also be used in protocols to address prostate prolapse and the soft surrounding tissues in men.

Future Harvests

Lady's mantle is a perennial plant that self-sows easily. Wildcrafting its aerial parts will not significantly affect future harvests.

HERBAL PREPARATIONS

Lady's mantle tea
Decoction
Drink ¼ cup as needed, or use topically as a skin wash or compress.

Lady's mantle tincture
1 part fresh flowers, leaves, and roots, chopped
2 parts menstruum (50 percent alcohol, 50 percent distilled water)
Take 15–25 drops as needed.

---

lemon balm

Melissa officinalis

PARTS USED flowers, leaves, stems

Lemon balm blossoms are loved by honey bees. Used traditionally as an apothecary herb, it is the perfect plant for calming overstressed nerves and increasing concentration.

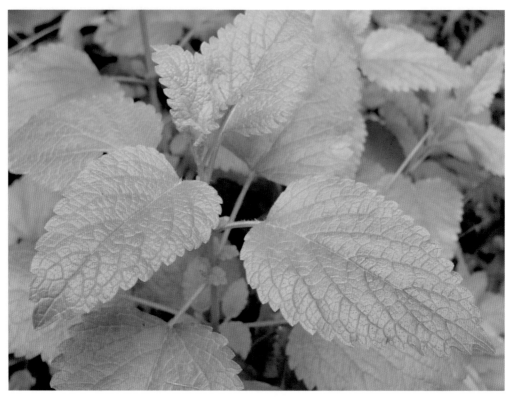

One of the best uses of lemon balm is as a tea to calm the nerves of any type-A or overachiever personality. It can also calm an upset stomach caused by nervous anxiety.

How to Identify

Lemon balm is an herbaceous perennial plant that grows 3–5 feet tall. A member of the mint family, lemon balm is easily identifiable by its scent and bright green, fuzzy, heart-shaped leaves that are arranged oppositely on square stems. The scent and taste of the plant is lemony, similar in aroma to citronella.

Lemon balm blooms in midsummer, producing whorled, white flower clusters that bear small nutlets in late summer.

Where, When, and How to Wildcraft

Look for lemon balm growing in dappled sun at the edges of the woods. It also frequently grows in gardens, where it can become

Chill Out: Decrease Your Stress with Aromatic Herbs

Stressed over work deadlines? Instead of reaching for that extra shot of espresso, reach for a cup of aromatic herbal tea to lift your spirits and calm your mind.

Lavender, lemon balm, mints, and rose are just a few plants with aromatic volatile oils that are uplifting and can provide a boost of energy without adding the extra stress on the system from caffeine. These herbs can also help clear a foggy head in the middle of a work-day, relieve tension, or soothe a headache caused by dramatic changes in weather.

At bedtime, if you're having trouble unwinding after a tough day, prepare a soothing tea blend of aromatic plants to help calm your mind.

Aromatic tea blend

Fresh or dry plant materials may be used in these ratios.

1 part lemon balm
1 part passionflower
1 part catnip
1 part elderflower
½ part holy basil (*Ocimum sanctum*)

1. Steep the blend in hot water for 2 minutes.
2. Strain the tea and sip it to promote restfulness and focus, and to soothe an anxious mind and stomach so you can sleep.

invasive. Wildcraft the tender leaves of spring for tea; they are most aromatic at that time, though the plant can be wildcrafted as needed throughout the growing season.

Wildcraft and bundle the stalks, and then dry them for tea. Or use the flowers, leaves, and stems fresh for a variety of preparations. Harvest the flowers in midsummer before the plant goes to seed in August; the plant is significantly drier to the touch after it produces seeds. In the fall, new leaves are as tender as spring leaves.

Medicinal Uses

One of the most traditional uses of lemon balm is as a calming tea. A strong, hot tea calms the nerves of any overachiever or type-A personality. Lemon balm tea is helpful for anyone who suffers from extreme stress in today's demanding society.

For an upset stomach caused by anxiety, use lemon balm in tea or in a bitters blend to relieve tension and stimulate digestion. Hot lemon balm tea can also be beneficial for colds and flus to relax tension resulting from fever and chills or excess coughing.

Lemon balm is also a wonderful antidote for sadness, melancholy, and heartache. Use a lemon balm honey infusion to sweeten teas, or swallow it by the spoonful to soothe a sore throat. Add catnip, chamomile, lavender, and rose petals to a cool infusion of lemon balm for a wonderful afternoon iced tea that tastes delicious with a splash of vodka and a fresh lemon wedge.

Future Harvests

Lemon balm is a voracious spreader. Its nutlets spread easily, and you can help propagate the spread of the plant by wildcrafting and planting the seeds in fall or starting them indoors. The plant can also be propagated by cuttings.

Lemon Balm Bitters for an Upset Tummy

In times of stress, the body slows the digestive process, and this can inhibit the proper uptake of core nutrients, leading to a different sort of malnutrition. Bitter herbs are a must for helping stagnant digestion that is symptomatic of excess stress.

Lemon balm or catnip also does wonders for soothing an anxious stomach. Blend it with aromatic herbs such as cinnamon or lavender in a tea or tincture.

Bitter foods (such as lemon balm, chamomile tea, dandelion leaves, and fennel) should be a main staple in our diets, and they can also be used as classic digestifs (similar to commercially made Campari or Angostura) or tinctured bitters. You can include a variety of plants in homemade bitters, such as aspen bark, cinnamon, fennel, and orange peel.

HERBAL PREPARATIONS

Lemon balm cold tea
Cold infusion
Drink 1 cup as needed.

Lemon balm hot tea
Hot infusion
Drink ¼ cup as needed.

Lemon balm tincture
1 part fresh flowers, leaves, and stems, chopped
2 parts menstruum (50 percent alcohol, 50 percent distilled water)
or
1 part dry flowers, leaves, and stems, chopped
4 parts menstruum (50 percent alcohol, 50 percent distilled water)
Take 25 drops as needed.

Lemon balm–infused honey
1 part fresh flowers and leaves, chopped
3 parts raw, unpasteurized honey
Use as needed.

Tilia species

basswood

PARTS USED bracts, flowers

In early summer, linden blossoms fill the air with a strong, sweet scent. Use them to create a soothing tea to calm upset nerves or for a fragrant, sweet syrup to use in sodas and cocktails.

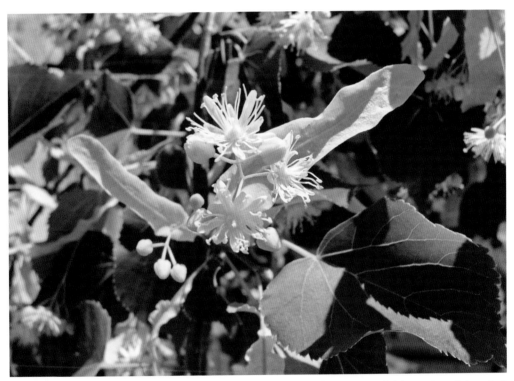

In early summer for about ten days, linden blossoms fill the air with a sweet and rich scent reminiscent of jasmine. Use your nose at this time of year to seek out these fragrant blossoms; they make a fine tea and cocktail syrup.

How to Identify

Linden trees can grow to heights of more than 80 feet. Their bark is dark gray and rough, with long, flat-topped ridges that look as though they have been smoothed with sandpaper. Leaves are heart-shaped, toothed, and slightly hairy on both sides. Flowers are white with five petals and long stamens; they bloom in clusters on branched bracts.

Where, When, and How to Wildcraft

Linden is well distributed across North America, and you'll find it growing in all temperate climates across the Midwest in mixed hardwood forests, particularly in river flood-plains, in rich, well-drained soil. It is also a common ornamental tree that is planted in neighborhoods and urban areas.

In early summer, the fragrance of linden flowers fills the air. Follow your nose to seek out these blossoms for use in tea and cocktail syrup. Honey bees will tell you when the linden blossoms are ready for wildcrafting: they flock to the trees to do their own wildcrafting of pollen and nectar. Take care as you gather the flowers, because you will be sharing space with these busy herbalists.

The flowers and bracts can both be harvested by trimming the entire bract and cluster from the branch. They will be sticky (and so will your hands), so wildcraft your harvest into a lint-free bag or basket.

Medicinal Uses

Tea made with fresh or dry linden flowers and bracts is deliciously sweet and fragrant, with a mild honeylike taste and a touch of jasmine fragrance. The mild tea is wonderful for soothing nerves. The fresh flowers and bracts can also be made into simple syrup with a similar honey-jasmine aroma that serves as a delicious base for homemade sodas, a sweetener for lemonade, or a cocktail ingredient. The syrup freezes well for winter use.

Future Harvests

Linden is a common tree that is distributed across the Midwest. Wildcrafting flowers in a quantity suitable for household use and consumption will not disturb plant distribution and future harvests.

HERBAL PREPARATIONS

Linden cold tea
Cold infusion
Drink 1 cup as needed.

Linden hot tea
Hot infusion
Drink ¼ cup as needed.

Linden tincture
1 part fresh bracts and flowers, chopped
2 parts menstruum (50 percent alcohol, 50 percent distilled water)
Take 25 drops as needed.

lobelia

Lobelia inflata
PARTS USED flowers, leaves, seedpods

Lobelia is a respiratory herb that is useful in easing congestion, facilitating expectoration, and soothing spasmodic coughing fits. It is also helpful in soothing muscles when included in massage oil.

How to Identify

Lobelia is an herbaceous perennial that is coarse and hairy and grows 2–3 feet tall. Its leaves are lance-shaped and alternate along the stem. Tiny, light blue, tubular flowers form in elongated clusters along racemes that emerge from the axils of the leaves. Inflated seedpods form in the late summer and fall, with oblong, brown seeds.

Where, When, and How to Wildcraft

Look for lobelia growing in moist, disturbed soils in roadsides, ditches, borrow pits, trails, and utility line clearings in deciduous forests. Wildcraft the flowers, leaves, and seedpods from the end of summer into early fall. They can be prepared fresh as a tincture or covered with oil and stored for later use.

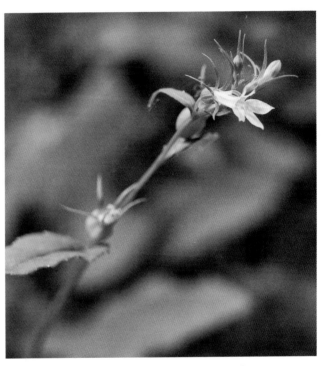

Tiny lobelia flowers bloom in late summer. As a relaxant expectorant, lobelia can help ease tight and constricted lung tissues and muscles to allow the lungs to move stuck mucus and subdue coughing spasms.

Medicinal Uses

Lobelia is commonly prepared as a tincture. As a relaxant, it can subdue coughing spasms and help ease tight and constricted lung tissues and muscles to enable the lungs to move stuck mucus and increase expectoration.

Use this herb to treat dry, barking coughs (including whooping cough) as well as damp, wet congestion related to acute pneumonia and pleurisy. For these conditions, lobelia can also be used in protocols along with other helpful respiratory herbs including butterfly weed, mullein, and wild cherry bark.

Prepare an antispasmodic massage oil with lobelia flowers, leaves, and seeds and use topically to soothe lung congestion. It is also helpful as a skeletal muscle relaxant and can help ease pain associated with sciatica and other back and neck pain.

Energetically, lobelia tincture in small-drop doses can help ease feelings of being stuck and dredging up the stuck energies or old memories and emotional wounds that may be holding a person back mentally. A massage oil of lobelia is also helpful in this case and is particularly useful in the practice of Maya abdominal massage for healing old traumatic injuries.

Future Harvests

Harvest wild lobelia mindfully, because habitat loss is affecting the distribution of this plant.

 Cautions, Concerns, and Considerations

The acrid nature of lobelia can elicit feelings of nausea. Contrary to some reports, the plant will not prove harmful if it is consumed appropriately and in small amounts.

HERBAL PREPARATIONS

Lobelia tincture
1 part fresh flowers and leaves, chopped
2 parts menstruum (95 percent alcohol,
    5 percent distilled water)
Take 10 drops as needed.

Lobelia-infused oil
1 part fresh flowers and leaves, chopped
2 parts oil
Use for massage.

---

lovage

Levisticum officinale

PARTS USED flowers, leaves, roots, seeds, stems

Spicy and aromatic, lovage is similar to angelica in flavor and smell.
Use the plant to soothe colds and flus, upset stomachs, and sore throats.

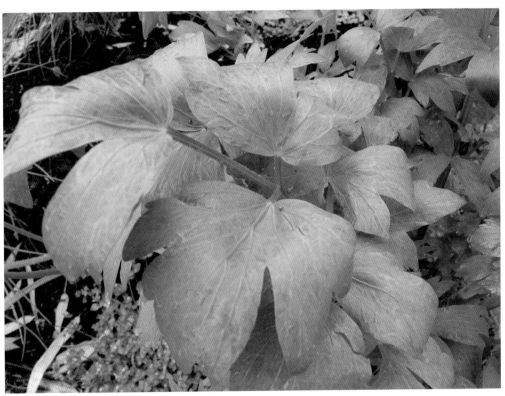

Lovage leaves are twice compound: each basal rosette of leaves and stems has a second set of leaflets. Lovage has notes similar in flavor and smell to osha and angelica.

How to Identify

Lovage is a perennial herbaceous plant that grows to 5 feet tall. The leaves are arranged oppositely on branching stems; they are twice compound, with lobed leaflets in sets of three that are serrated, smooth, and green. Lovage flowers in yellow-green umbels in late June. By late summer, small, oval, and brownish seeds are produced. The root is fleshy and light brown in color. When crushed, the entire plant smells similar to celery or angelica.

Where, When, and How to Wildcraft

Lovage prefers moist or damp soil. It grows along hedgerows or in gardens as a weed. Wildcraft the roots in early spring before the plant begins to branch out and flower.

Prepare the roots fresh, or dry them for later use. Wildcraft the flowers, leaves, seeds, and stems in summer.

Medicinal Uses

A relative of angelica, lovage is not a replacement for angelica but can be used in similar ways. Chew the highly aromatic seeds to clear sinuses and soothe an upset stomach. Or chew them when you notice a cold coming on. The flavors are warming and drying.

Make a warming, aromatic tea from fresh or dry roots and leaves; flavor the tea with hyssop and sweeten it with honey. Savor the tea to relieve a chill from cold, damp weather, or to soothe a stomachache or damp cough. Prepare a tincture of fresh or dry leaves, roots, and seeds to use similarly.

Mix dried roots with honey for a chewy lozenge to soothe an upset stomach or for a soothing throat remedy. Chop fresh stalks and coat them in cane sugar to offer for stomachaches as a carminative herb. Infuse the aerial parts, roots, and seeds in honey to add to tea, or take it medicinally by the spoonful to soothe a sore throat.

Future Harvests

Lovage is a perennial and self-sows easily. Wildcrafting moderate amounts of the plant will not significantly affect future harvests.

 Cautions, Concerns, and Considerations

The appearance of the lovage plant is similar to that of another member of the Apiaceae— poison hemlock (*Conium maculatum*). If there is any doubt about the plant, do not handle it without wearing gloves, because the toxicity of poison hemlock can be absorbed through the skin. Certainly do not taste the plant if you are unsure! Seek an experienced herbalist or botanist who can help you confirm the plant's identification. Once you do learn the plant's chief identifiers and are able to identify it correctly, your wildcrafted lovage will be a valuable addition to your apothecary and spice cabinets.

HERBAL PREPARATIONS

Lovage tea
Infusion
Drink ½ cup as needed.

Lovage tincture
1 part fresh flowers, leaves, roots, seeds, and
  stems, chopped
2 parts menstruum (95 percent alcohol,
  5 percent distilled water)
Take 10–15 drops as needed.

Lovage-infused honey
1 part fresh flowers and leaves, chopped
3 parts raw, unpasteurized honey
Use as needed.

---

lungwort

Pulmonaria officinalis
Jerusalem cowslip
PARTS USED flowers, leaves

A cousin of borage and comfrey, lungwort can be used in a relaxing tea that calms nerves, soothes coughs, and relieves congestion.

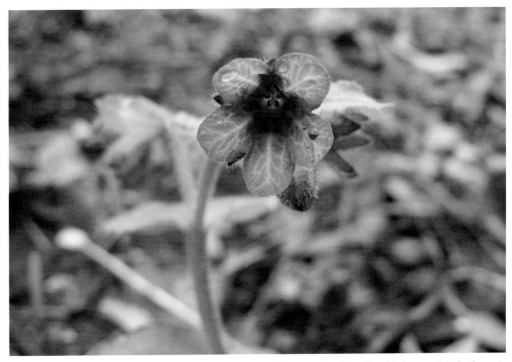

Lungwort flowers are red or pink at first and later turn to blue-purple when the pH changes inside the petals. The fresh leaves and flowers can be prepared similarly to borage as a cool infusion for a soothing tea.

How to Identify

Lungwort is a small evergreen perennial herb. The fuzzy leaves are green, heart-shaped, and pointed, and they grow alternately along the stem. Leaves usually have rounded and often sharply defined white or pale green patches. The plant blooms in early May with clusters of five-petaled flowers that begin as pink and then change to a blue-purple color.

Where, When, and How to Wildcraft

Look for lungwort in dappled shade in the woods. In the early spring, it pushes through the ground at the end of April, and mature leaves, best for wildcrafting, are available for harvest by early May. Wildcraft flowers and leaves in spring. Use them fresh or dry them for later use.

Medicinal Uses

Lungwort has cooling and mucilaginous properties similar to those of its cousins borage and comfrey. The fresh leaves and flowers of lungwort can be prepared similarly to borage as a cool infusion for tea. As a nerve tonic, add lemon balm to the tea and sweeten it with honey.

Traditionally, lungwort leaves have been used to soothe hot, dry respiratory congestion and barking coughs. Combine lungwort leaf tea with coltsfoot or mullein and sweeten with honey to relieve congestion. Add wild cherry bark to a cool infusion of lungwort to help ease spasmodic coughing.

Future Harvests

Lungwort frequently escapes from cultivation and self-sows well. It can easily be cultivated into a woodland permaculture space.

Harvest leaves sparingly to avoid affecting future harvests.

Cautions, Concerns, and Considerations

There is a great deal of discussion in the herbal community regarding the safety of lungwort when used internally based on the presence of alkaloids that could be potentially toxic to the liver. Although the debate against lungwort's use is widely unsubstantiated, it is always prudent, if in doubt, to choose to work with another herb.

HERBAL PREPARATIONS

Lungwort tea
Infusion
Drink ¼ cup as needed.

---

maitake

Grifola frondosa
hen of the woods
PARTS USED fruiting body

High in nutrients and beneficial to the immune system, maitake is an important medicinal mushroom to use as a functional food and medicine in the apothecary.

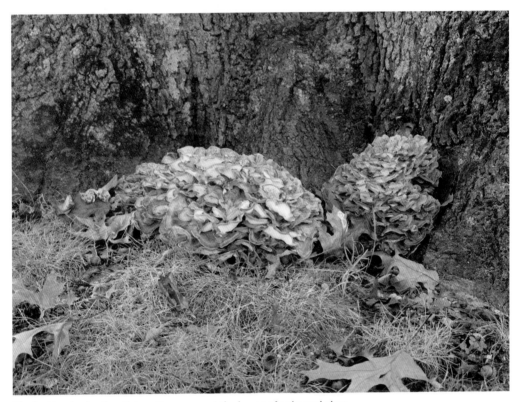

The fruiting body of maitake often grows at the bases of oaks and elms.

How to Identify

Maitake is a polypore, a bracket fungus in which white spores are expelled through fine pores on the underside of the fungus. This parasitic fungus grows at the bases of dying oaks and elms. The compact, clustered rosette of overlapping gray-white or brown fronds feed off the roots and bases of the trees, causing a white rot of the wood.

Where, When, and How to Wildcraft

Look for the folded and lobed fruiting body growing in woodlands at the bases of dying oaks and elms in September. Carefully cut away the upper portion of the maitake, taking care not to remove the entire fungus from the tree. Prepare it fresh or dry it for use across the seasons.

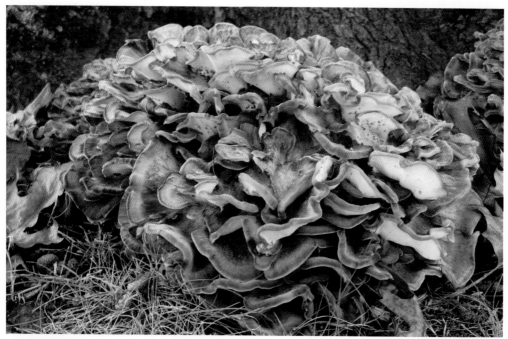

Maitake first and foremost is an important functional food that can offer significant nutrition to the body including B vitamins, vitamin D, potassium, plant proteins, and carbohydrates that can nourish the immune system.

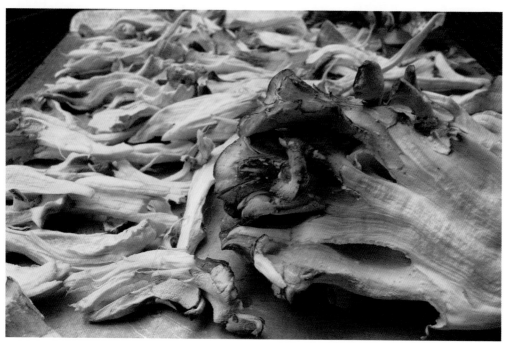

Maitake sliced and prepared for drying. Dried maitake is used for tea and broths.

Medicinal Uses

Maitake first and foremost is an important functional food that can offer significant nutrition to the body, including vitamins D and B complex, potassium, plant proteins, and carbohydrates that can nourish the immune system. It is delicious in sautés and stir-fries or on its own, cooked in butter.

Medicinally, dried maitake can be prepared as a decoction for tea to concentrate its properties. It is a tasty addition to broths, along with chaga, nettle, oatstraw, red clover, and reishi, for a mineral-dense infusion that can nourish the immune system.

Future Harvests

To ensure future harvestability, carefully cut away part of the fungus, rather than taking all of it.

HERBAL PREPARATIONS

Maitake tea
Decoction
Drink 1 cup per day.

meadowsweet

Filipendula ulmaria
PARTS USED flowers

Aromatic and astringent meadowsweet works well as an anti-inflammatory. It is a valuable medicine to aid in stomach distress and a popular musculoskeletal remedy for aches and pains.

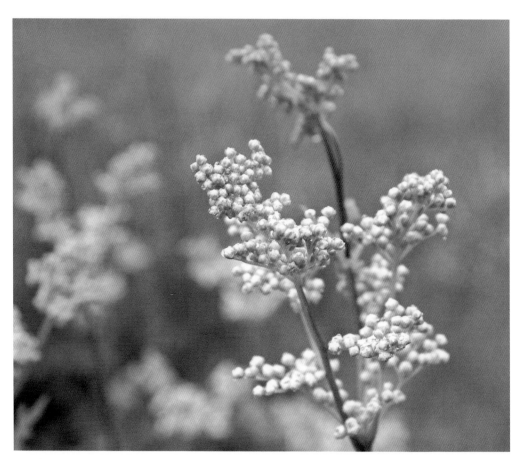

Meadowsweet is aromatic and astringent and works well as an anti-inflammatory. Its delicate flowers bloom throughout the summer.

How to Identify

Meadowsweet is a perennial shrub that grows 3–6 feet tall, with branching, thin stems that are often purple in color. Leaves are dark green, pinnately compound, with 3–7 serrated leaflets. Meadowsweet flowers in June, producing creamy white to yellowish umbels of flowers with a slight musky aroma.

Where, When, and How to Wildcraft

Look for meadowsweet growing wild in damp meadows and in landscape plantings. Wildcraft the flowers when the plant is dry and in full bloom in early summer. Process the blossoms immediately to use fresh or lay the umbels flat to dry for later use.

Medicinal Uses

For stomach distress, blend meadowsweet into a bitters formula with other herbs such as lemon balm and ceanothus to help soothe indigestion. Add it to herbal protocols to help soothe stomach ulcers. It works well in combination with relaxant herbs such as chamomile and tissue-healing herbs such as marshmallow, plantain, and slippery elm.

As an herb useful in musculoskeletal injuries, meadowsweet can help soothe muscle injuries and ease arthritic and rheumatic pain in the joints and soft tissues. Infuse meadowsweet flowers in oil to use for massage or prepare them in a balm.

Meadowsweet blends well with other anti-inflammatory herbs such as clove and turmeric and musculoskeletal herbs such as goldenrod. These herbal combinations can also be prepared as a tincture and applied topically to muscles and joints as a liniment. They are particularly helpful for athletes who suffer regular injury or for those who want to relieve pain from arthritis or fibromyalgia.

Meadowsweet flowers can also be ground into a powder and blended with Epsom salts for a relaxing post-workout bath.

Future Harvests

Meadowsweet is a hardy perennial plant, and wildcrafting the flowers in moderation will do little to affect future harvests.

HERBAL PREPARATIONS

Meadowsweet tea
Infusion
Drink ¼ cup as needed, or use topically as a wash or compress.

Meadowsweet tincture
1 part fresh flowers
2 parts menstruum (50 percent alcohol, 50 percent distilled water)
or
1 part dry flowers
4 parts menstruum (50 percent alcohol, 50 percent distilled water)
Take 15–20 drops as needed, or use topically as a liniment.

Meadowsweet-infused oil
1 part fresh flowers
2 parts oil
Use for massage.

---

motherwort

Leonurus cardiaca
PARTS USED flowers, leaves

Motherwort is a useful apothecary herb to help soothe nervous tensions and anxiety. It's a perfect medicinal herb for new moms or overworked professionals.

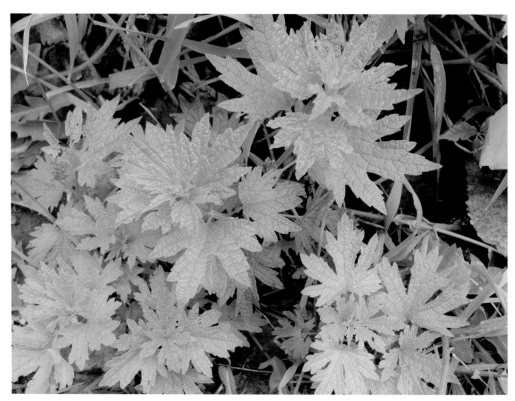

Motherwort can be mixed with other herbs, especially aromatics like chamomile, lavender, and lemon balm, to round out the flavor and make a nice relaxant tea.

How to Identify

Motherwort is a biennial plant in the mint family. The first-year leaves grow in a basal rosette; they are deep green, mostly palmate, and deeply lobed with usually five lobes, with some variations. Second-year leaves grow in an opposite arrangement up the square stem. They are narrow and entire, often trilobed. Leaf undersides have variable-length hairs.

The wooly blossoms appear in July and are favorites of honey bees. Showy pinkish to white flower clusters grow in whorls along the stem. The plant has a pungent odor and a very bitter taste.

Where, When, and How to Wildcraft

Motherwort tolerates many soil conditions and grows in open fields, along trails, in

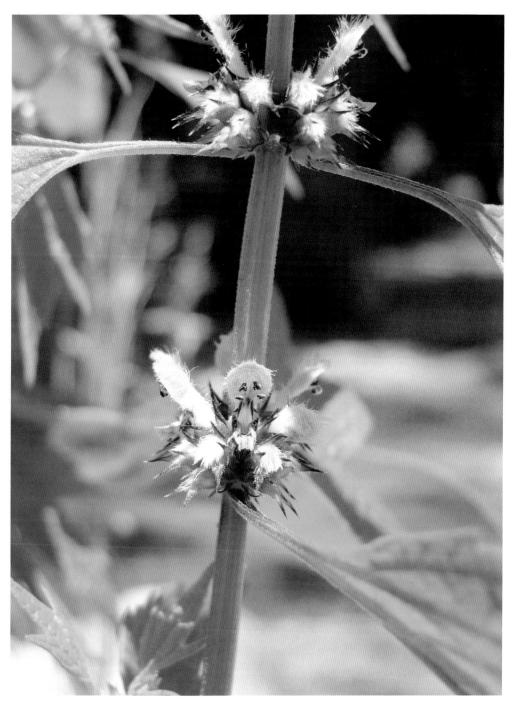

For a relaxant massage oil good for new mothers, motherwort leaves and flowers can be blended with violet leaves and flowers and dandelion flowers. This makes for a good lymphatic breast massage oil as well as stomach massage oil.

disturbed areas, and in garden beds, where it is usually identified as a weed. Wildcraft the new leaves of motherwort in early spring; they will be strongly bitter. Collect the leaves on a dry day, selecting those that are free of dust and debris. Dry them on screens for later use, or use them fresh in a tea or massage oil. Wildcraft the flowers during their bloom time in July to use fresh in a tincture or an oil infusion.

Medicinal Uses

Motherwort is used to soothe nervous tension and anxiety, especially for those who tend to overthink. Use it in a tea with other herbs, especially aromatics such as chamomile, lavender, and lemon balm, to round out the flavor and make a relaxant beverage, sweetened with honey. It is a good herb to integrate into a support protocol for a cigarette-cessation plan, because the herb can help calm the anxiety that comes from nicotine withdrawal.

Motherwort can also be extracted into vodka or brandy to make a bitters blend. Sweeten the blend with honey to make an elixir to add to tea or use in herbal cocktails—think lavender martini with a dash of motherwort bitters.

For a relaxant massage oil for new mothers, make an infusion blend of motherwort leaves and flowers, dandelion flowers, and violet flowers and leaves. This is a good lymphatic breast massage oil and a stomach massage oil that works well in combination with Maya abdominal massage techniques.

Future Harvests

Motherwort is a hardy biennial plant that grows nearly everywhere. It propagates prolifically from seed and is easily transplanted. Wildcrafting basal leaves and flower spikes will not significantly impact future harvests.

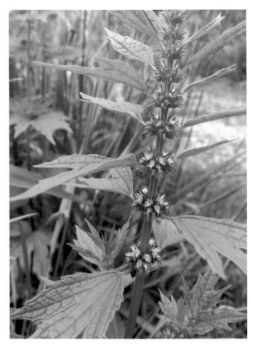

Flowers grow in whorls along the leaf axils.

HERBAL PREPARATIONS

Motherwort tea
Infusion
Drink ¼ cup as needed.

Motherwort tincture
1 part fresh flowers and leaves, chopped
2 parts menstruum (50 percent alcohol, 50 percent distilled water)
Take 25 drops as needed.

Motherwort-infused oil
1 part fresh flowers and leaves, chopped
2 parts oil
Use for massage.

Motherwort-infused honey
1 part fresh flowers and leaves, chopped
3 parts raw, unpasteurized honey
Use as needed.

mullein

Verbascum thapsus

PARTS USED flowers, leaves, roots

From roots to flowers, the entire mullein plant can be used in a multitude of ways in remedies for respiratory health, lymphatic support, and musculoskeletal complaints.

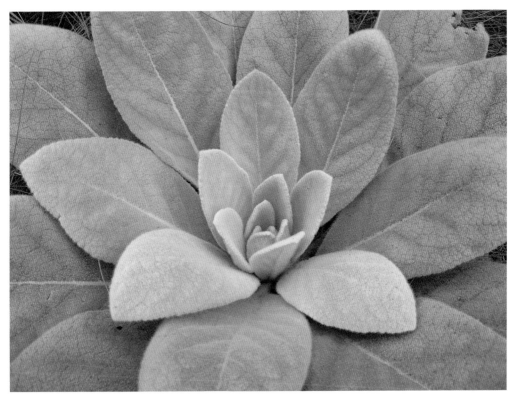

Mullein tea, and also the root as a plant extract, can noticeably reduce acute inflammation of joint injuries. Back out of whack? Creaky joints? Try a few quarts of mullein tea.

How to Identify

Mullein is a biennial plant, identifiable by the long, ovate, and markedly hairy basal leaves of the grayish green rosette in the first year of growth. In the second year, mullein sends up a flower stalk that can grow to 7 feet or taller, giving way to a showy flower spike of yellow blossoms that bloom until late summer.

Mullein root is small and spindly, compared to the size of the basal rosette and the flowering stalk. It is gray-white in color with an earthy mineral flavor.

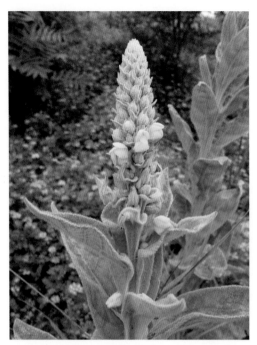
You can use the entire mullein plant as medicine for musculoskeletal injuries, respiratory issues, and lymphatic health.

Where, When, and How to Wildcraft

Look for mullein growing abundantly in full sun in open fields, urban lots, and old pastures, and alongside highways—any place where the soil is rocky and of poor quality. Mullein withers under wet and damp conditions, so it is best to wildcraft it on a clear, dry, and sunny day.

Wildcraft mullein leaves starting in the first year of growth. Cut them from the rosette with a small knife or kitchen shears. Although you can harvest the leaves at any time of year, be sure to choose leaves that have not been significantly damaged by insects, which occurs frequently late in the growing season. Dry the leaves in a bundle or chop them roughly and dry them on a screen to use for tea.

If you are harvesting the plant roots, the entire rosette and roots can be wildcrafted at the same time throughout the season, but take care to remove the root from the soil and do not get sand on the hairy leaves—removing sand and soil will be nearly impossible, particularly because the hairy leaves do not wash well. If you're preserving the root, clean it fully and include the fine hairs as well as the crown. Chop and dry it in a dehydrator or make a plant extract using grain alcohol.

The flowers, which begin to bloom in midsummer, are tedious to wildcraft, because you must hand pick each one. Children are good helpers in this case. The blooms are beautiful and a delight to seek out. Dry them on a screen or preserve them in oil or grain alcohol to use later.

Medicinal Uses

Mullein is a great plant to wildcraft, because it is useful for the home apothecary as well as for a field medicine to treat musculoskeletal injuries, respiratory issues, and lymphatic health.

Mullein leaf is traditionally used as a relaxant herb to relieve chest and lung congestion. Mullein tea dries a wet cough and helps calm spasmodic coughing. In preparing the leaf tea, strain it through a coffee filter to remove the fine hairs, which can irritate throat tissues. Add honey to make it especially soothing.

Prepare fresh mullein flowers preserved in a bit of olive oil (with garlic) to soothe sinus congestion that affects the ear and causes earache. This homemade preparation is significantly better (and cheaper) than the commercial products available at health food stores.

Mullein's fine hairs can aggravate the skin, but this quality is helpful as a field medicine and makes a good poultice for inflamed joints or bursitis injuries that may flare up on the trail. The tea, and also the root as a plant extract, can noticeably reduce acute inflammation of joint injuries caused by a trauma or misalignment.

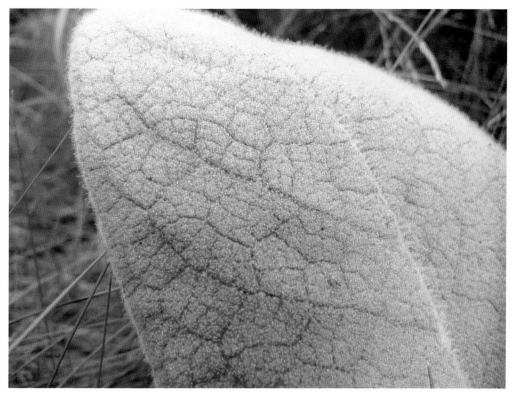

Mullein leaf is most known for its use as a relaxant herb for chest and lung congestion. The tea dries a wet cough and helps calm spasmodic coughing.

Future Harvests

Mullein is a common plant. Even though the plant produces thousands of seeds, it is difficult to propagate by seed because sometimes the germination rate is nil. It grows where it wishes.

 Cautions, Concerns, and Considerations

Do not use the mullein leaf as toilet paper in the field, because its fine hairs aggravate tender membranes. Consider yourself warned!

HERBAL PREPARATIONS

Mullein tea
Decoction
Drink 2 cups as needed.

Mullein tincture
1 part fresh flowers, leaves, and roots, chopped
2 parts menstruum (50 percent alcohol, 50 percent distilled water)
Take 10–15 drops, 3 to 5 times per day.

Mullein-infused oil
1 part fresh flowers and leaves, chopped
2 parts oil
Use for massage.

nettle

Urtica dioica
itchweed, stinging nettle
PARTS USED leaves, seeds

Nettle is a nourishing and functional herb that doubles as a food and a medicine. It offers minerals and is tonifying for the body. The sting of the nettle can also be medicinal by helping restore sensation to areas of the body that are deadened from nerve damage or that suffer from ghost pain.

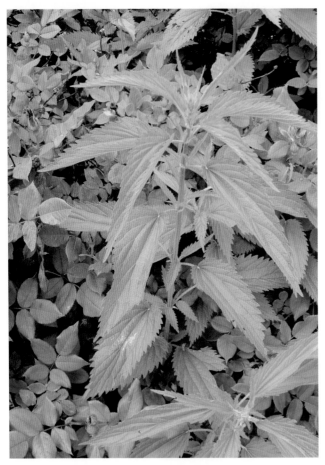

Nettles have great virtues as a nutritional food, which is especially important for the convalescing person. Nettles are nutrient dense—rich in vitamins C and A, calcium, magnesium, zinc, iron, cobalt, copper, potassium, B-complex vitamins, and even protein—and are high in chlorophyll.

How to Identify

Nettle is a perennial plant that grows to 8 feet tall in rich, nutrient-dense soil. Its oppositely arranged leaves are oblong, dark green on top and lighter green underneath, roughly toothed, and deeply veined. Flowers are tiny, greenish or brownish in color, and grow in a dense inflorescence near the stop of the stem.

Stinging hairs occur up and down the plant's stems and on the undersides of the leaves. These fine, sharp, hollow hairs are filled with formic acid, which is released when they pierce or break and scratch the skin. A nettle sting is similar to a bee sting, although not quite as painful. Contacting the nettle causes an immediate itching sensation and a skin rash. The sensation is similar to the feeling you might get if you rubbed fiberglass on your skin.

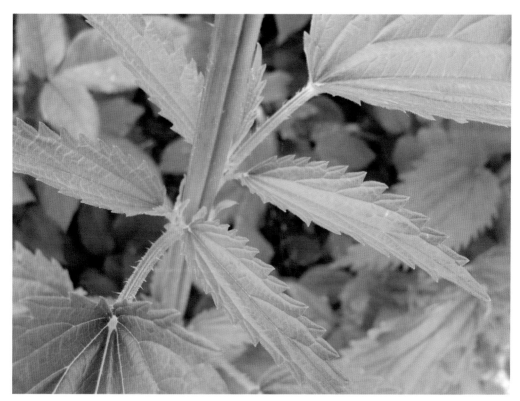

One of nettle's chief identifiers is its sting. Stinging nettle has fine, sharp, hollow hairs filled with formic acid that can pierce or break and scratch the skin, injecting or releasing the acid. The sting dissipates when the leaves are cooked or dried.

Where, When, and How to Wildcraft

Look for nettle in the spring (April to June) or late fall (October or November) in areas with nitrogen-rich, damp soil. You'll often find it growing adjacent to rivers, streams, lakes, springs, ditches, wetlands, and drainage areas.

Wearing gloves, pick the tender leaves and stems in early spring and late fall, both before and after the plant goes to seed. Wildcraft the seeds that are produced in late fall. Because the stems can get very tough and woody as the plant ages, harvest plants with smaller, more tender stems, or harvest leaves earlier in the spring season when they are most delicious. Collect the upper stalks when they reach about 18 inches tall; this is a great size to bundle and dry in a protected spot. Otherwise, chop the leaves and stems for drying or freezing, or use them fresh in cooked dishes. The nettle sting dissipates upon cooking or drying.

To dry nettles, spread chopped or whole plants onto racks (window screens are great for this task) and let everything dry completely before storing it in glass jars. If the plant material is not completely dry before storage, it can mold.

Medicinal Uses

Nettle has great virtues as a nutritional food, especially important for the convalescing person. Nettles are very nutrient-dense and rich in vitamins C, A, and B complex; calcium; magnesium; zinc; iron; cobalt;

Mineral-Dense, Plant-Based Broths

Is it broth or stock? There is much banter among culinary professionals regarding the difference between the two. I consider stock, which is made from bones, meat, and soft tissue, and sometimes prepared with herbs and veggies, a key staple in the kitchen. I consider broth the final preparation that is actually served at the table. I say *po-tay-to*, you say *po-tah-to*.

As an herbalist, I focus on making broths with nutritive benefits that come from cooking animal bones, soft connective tissue, plants, and mushrooms. I frequently add nutritive herbs and medicinal plants such as astragalus, burdock, horsetail, nettle, oatstraw, red clover, seaweed, and wildcrafted medicinal mushrooms such as chaga, maitake, reishi, and shitake. Antioxidant-rich mushrooms support cellular repair with their powerful polysaccharides.

Stock made with animal bones and connective tissues is packed with collagen and gelatin, which are necessary building blocks for human tissue rebuilding and repair. I always recommend making animal-based broths for convalescing, but I have many clients who prefer to have plant-based recipes. This is my version of a plant-powered vegan stock that is high in bioavailable minerals such as calcium, magnesium, potassium, and silica.

Wild plant–powered vegan stock

In case of gluten intolerance, remove the oatstraw and increase the nettle, red clover, and raspberry leaf.

About 2 cups dry herbs mix
(mix and match as you wish):
   astragalus root (2 sticks)
   bull kelp seaweed
   dry burdock root
   horsetail (if suffering from muscle
      tissue injury)
   jujube (*Ziziphus jujube*) fruit
   nettle
   oatstraw
   raspberry leaf
   red clover
   wolfberries (goji berries)
1 cup dry mushrooms of choice, or
      3 tablespoons of powdered mush-
      rooms (mix and match as you wish):
   chaga
   maitake
   shitake
   reishi

1. Boil the herbal mixture and mush-rooms in 4 quarts of water for 20 minutes.
2. Don't be concerned about sim-mering versus boiling. In this case, we want a mineral extraction from the plant material, and you cannot destroy minerals with heat because they are an earth's element. A long cooking (extraction) time is needed to extract the minerals.
3. Strain and store the liquid in jars or containers and refrigerate it for up to 2 days, or it can be frozen for later use. This stock is excel-lent when used for chilled ice tea, warmed in a mug, added to smoothies (in place of the water), or used as a vegan base for soups and other dishes.

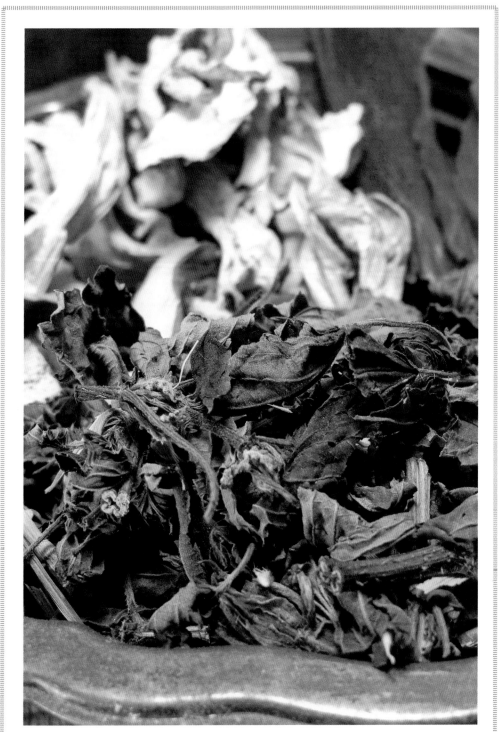

Use dry nettle with maitake and hand-harvested seaweed to create mineral-dense teas and herb-fortified bone broths.

copper; potassium; and even protein. They are extremely high in chlorophyll.

Topically, nettle is used to treat bodily areas of nerve damage or areas that experience ghost pain. The nettle's sting can stimulate a nervous system response and help restore sensation. Include a tincture of nettle seed in protocols for kidney and urinary tract weakness and to support male fertility.

Boil the leaves to speed up the mineral extraction time, or let them steep overnight. Other herbs that work well in a nourishing infusion include oatstraw and red clover. Enjoy the blend as a warm or iced tea, or use it as a vegan broth for soups, rice, and pasta.

The plant has a neutral green flavor, similar to that of spinach, and it is equally versatile in recipes. In comparison to other green superfoods, nettle flavor knocks it out of the park! Enjoy the dried leaves year-round, adding them to soups and brewing them as a mineral-dense beverage. Infusing nettle in vinegar extracts the minerals from the plant, and this is a great addition to the pantry to use in salad dressings and add mineral density to foods.

Future Harvests

Nettle is a rapidly growing perennial that thrives in moist areas. Wildcraft upper stalks, stems, and leaves, but let much of the plant remain intact for photosynthesis to occur and to ensure next season's growth.

 ### Cautions, Concerns, and Considerations

Wear harvesting gloves and long pants to minimize the potential for skin irritation from the nettle's sting. Use gloves when processing nettle in the kitchen, too. The severity and length of the irritation depends on the individual, but immediately rinsing the area with cold water is a good first step. The juice of the plant can neutralize its sting; crushed dock leaves or jewelweed stalks can also take the sting away. Excess exposure to the formic acid can cause redness and welts on the skin that can last up to 36 hours. Drying or cooking the plant will cause the formic acid to dissipate.

Because nettle thrives in damp soils along river and stream banks, know the area from which you are harvesting and its history of use. Avoid areas adjacent to or downstream from large factories and farms to avoid harvesting contaminated plants.

HERBAL PREPARATIONS

Nettle tea
Decoction
Drink 2 cups per day.

Nettle tincture
1 part fresh leaves, chopped
2 parts menstruum (50 percent alcohol, 50 percent distilled water)
or
1 part dry leaves, chopped
4 parts menstruum (50 percent alcohol, 50 percent distilled water)
Take 15–20 drops per day.

Nettle-infused vinegar
1 part fresh leaves, chopped
3 parts raw apple cider vinegar
Take 2–3 tablespoons per day.

New England aster

Symphyotrichum novae-angliae
PARTS USED flowers, leaves

New England aster is a useful herb to have on hand for springtime allergies. This aromatic and astringent plant helps dry up dripping sinuses caused by hay fever or animal dander allergies.

How to Identify

New England aster is a clumping perennial that grows 4–6 feet tall. The entire plant is slightly hairy and dry to the touch. Its ovate leaves are slender, 3–4 inches long, and grow alternately on the stem.

In the fall, showy blossoms emerge, with pink to dark purple rays of flowers with yellow to golden centers. The entire plant is aromatic, resinous, and sticky to the touch when crushed. It is slightly astringent on the tongue, making the mouth feel dry.

Where, When, and How to Wildcraft

You'll find New England aster growing throughout the Midwest in sunny, open, moist fields and wetland areas. It thrives in ditches and stream beds. After flowers bloom in late summer, they will be full of pollinators on sunny days. Harvest blossoms in the full sun.

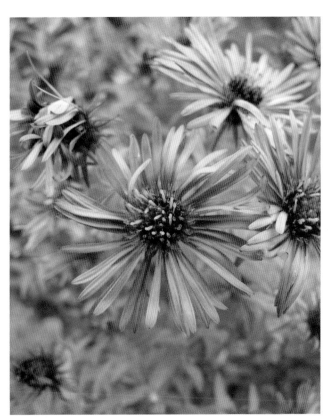

New England aster is an aromatic and astringent plant that is useful in helping dry up leaking and dripping sinuses caused by hay fever or sensitivity to cats.

Depending on the size of the stand, entire plant stalks can be wildcrafted in the fall. Strip the flowers and leaves from the stems and dry them for later use, or use them fresh in the kitchen.

After harvesting, the flowers will quickly become puffy seed balls, which can be frustrating to manage if you are trying to dry them for tea. Cover the bundled stalks loosely with a paper bag to help contain the seed fluff while they dry.

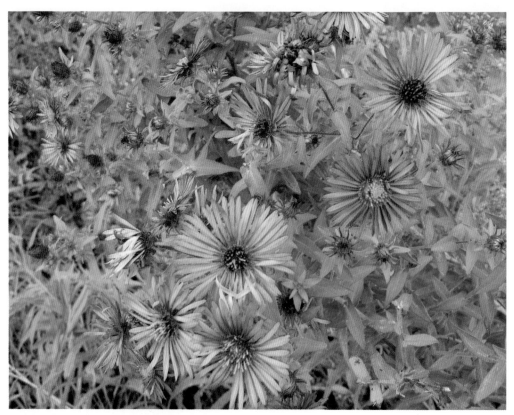

New England aster's delicate blooms are abundant in September and attract many pollinators.

Medicinal Uses

Prepare New England aster leaves and flowers as a hot tea or as a plant tincture made from glycerin or grain spirits. It blends well with ground ivy, goldenrod, mullein, and nettle.

To balance the drying effect of the plant on the throat and lungs, add raw honey to the preparation to soothe the mucosa. Even better, infuse the aromatic fresh plant into local raw honey, strain, and then keep it on hand to add to tea.

Future Harvests

New England aster is widely distributed and is a wonderful plant to attract pollinators. Collect plants in moderation to promote self-seeding and continued harvesting of this showy perennial.

HERBAL PREPARATIONS

New England aster tea
Infusion
Drink ¼ cup as needed.

New England aster tincture
1 part fresh flowers and leaves, chopped
2 parts menstruum (95 percent alcohol, 5 percent distilled water)
Take 10–15 drops as needed.

New England aster–infused honey
1 part fresh flowers and leaves, chopped
3 parts raw, unpasteurized honey
Use as needed.

Quercus species
red oak (*Q. rubra*), white oak (*Q. alba*)
PARTS USED inner and outer bark, leaves

Oak bark is used as an astringent medicine for topical wound care.

How to Identify

Red oaks are identifiable by their dark red-dish gray bark that is heavily ridged. Leaves alternate along the stem and are clustered at the terminal bud. They are obovate to oblong, 5–10 inches long and 4–6 inches wide, with seven to nine pointed lobes. Mature red oaks can grow to 90 feet or more and may live up to 500 years. Bitter-tasting acorns emerge in late summer and early fall.

White oaks have light gray bark that is shallow ridged. In spring, young leaves are silvery pink and covered with soft down. Leaves grow alternately, are 5–8 inches long and 3–4 inches wide, and have a glossy green upper surface. Obovate or oblong, they usually have seven rounded lobes. Mature white oaks can grow to 100 feet tall and live for up to 300 years. Acorns emerge in late summer and early fall.

To discern between the two types of oaks, remember that red oaks have pointed-lobed leaves and white oaks have round-lobed leaves. Leaves of both can be deeply lobed or have no lobes, however. Some brown, dead leaves may remain on both species throughout winter until very early spring when the trees begin to produce buds.

Where, When, and How to Wildcraft

Both red and white oaks are tolerant of a variety of soils and growing conditions and are well

For a topical wash, make an infusion of dry leaves or oak bark. Strain and use topically to clean and astringe weepy wounds including fungal infections and poison ivy.

distributed across the Midwest in both forests and urban settings. Gather the inner and outer bark and dry leaves across the seasons to use for medicine. Dry bark pieces in the sun and store them in a sealed container.

Medicinal Uses

For a topical wash, make a decoction of the dry leaves or bark, strain, and use topically to clean and astringe weepy wounds, including fungal infections and poison ivy rashes. Sprinkle finely powdered dried inner bark on external wounds to prevent infection and to soothe, reduce swelling, and strengthen tissues.

Future Harvests

Oaks are widespread across the Midwest and have not yet been threatened by Sudden Oak Death (caused by the pathogen *Phytophthora ramorum*), which is ravaging California and Oregon trees, but oak wilt (caused by the fungus *Ceratocystis fagacearum*) is a concern in the Midwest. Habitat loss is also an issue for our large hardwoods. Gathering the leaves and bark in a sustainable way will not significantly affect future harvests.

HERBAL PREPARATIONS

Oak leaf or bark tea
Decoction
Use topically for astringent wound wash.

Oregon grape

Mahonia aquifolium
PARTS USED leaves, rhizomes

Oregon grape has an important role in the herbal apothecary as a helpful bitters that can support digestion, and it works as an antibacterial for septic infections and topical wounds.

How to Identify

Oregon grape is a perennial shrub that grows 2–5 feet tall. It is a branching plant with thick stems and compound pinnate leaves 12 inches long, with bright green, shiny, and spiny leaflets that resemble holly leaves.

Bright yellow flower clusters bloom on the branch terminals in early spring and develop into dark blue berries in late summer. The leaves turn a bright red color in late fall and winter. The creeping rhizomes are yellow-brown and woody.

Where, When and How to Wildcraft

Oregon grape prefers moist, well-drained soil and full sun. In the Midwest, it is most often grown in gardens as a cultivated ornamental plant.

Harvest the leaves across the season to use fresh or dry them for later use. Gather the rhizomes of the plant in early spring and in late fall, after the plant has gone dormant. Take care to select the outer lateral rhizomes to avoid disturbing future growth. Use the small rhizomes fresh or dry them for tea or tincture. Remove the outer bark of larger rhizomes before drying or preparing them as a tincture or tea.

Medicinal Uses

Oregon grape is very astringent and is used to help dry, tighten, and tone tissues and wounds that are infected or inflamed.

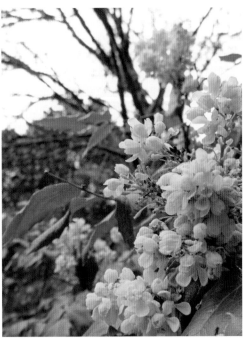

Oregon grape is very astringent and can be useful in helping dry, tighten, and tone tissues and wounds that may be affected by infection or inflammation.

Prepare a topical wash with the leaves or root bark, or dilute the tincture in water to use topically to clean and dry up wet, weepy wounds such as poison ivy rashes.

Oregon grape is a markedly bitter herb that helps stimulate damp and sluggish digestion. It also serves as an overall digestive tonic to assist with assimilation (nutrient uptake) and elimination. It supports the liver by stimulating bile production, which in turn can help with digestion and assimilation of fats.

Although Oregon grape can be used alone as a tea or tincture, its bitter flavor is more palatable when it is mixed with other herbs. For both flavor and effectiveness, Oregon grape blends well with warming aromatics such as angelica as well as other digestive herbs such as burdock root and dandelion root and lymphatic herbs such as ceanothus.

Adding an aromatic and bitter nervine tonic such as lemon balm is useful for stomach ailments and stagnant digestion related to nervous tension. These blends can help balance the digestive system to support hormone balance and stabilize insulin levels, and they can be used to clear skin conditions such as chronic eczema.

The high berberine content in Oregon grape makes it effective as a broad-spectrum antimicrobial herb for a tincture or tea (especially when used as a topical wound wash) in protocols to address septic infections, including staph infections.

Future Harvests

Although Oregon grape is native to western North America, it has been widely planted in the Midwest as an ornamental plant. Wild populations of the plant are considered rare here. The good news is that it is readily available from nurseries if you want to grow your own. Harvest the lateral rhizomes carefully to avoid disturbing the main rhizomes and ensure future harvests. The plant is drought- and cold-tolerant and can be added into a permaculture plan for cultivation.

HERBAL PREPARATIONS

Oregon grape tea
Decoction
Drink ¼ cup as needed, or use topically as a wound wash.

Oregon grape tincture
1 part fresh rhizomes, chopped
2 parts menstruum (50 percent alcohol, 50 percent distilled water)
or
1 part dry rhizomes, chopped
4 parts menstruum (50 percent alcohol, 50 percent distilled water)
Take 15–20 drops as needed.

ox-eye daisy

Leucanthemum vulgare
PARTS USED flowers, leaves

The showy ox-eye daisy is a helpful herb to use as a wound care remedy and for seasonal allergy relief. Ox-eye daisy is an astringent, slightly aromatic, bitter, and drying herb.

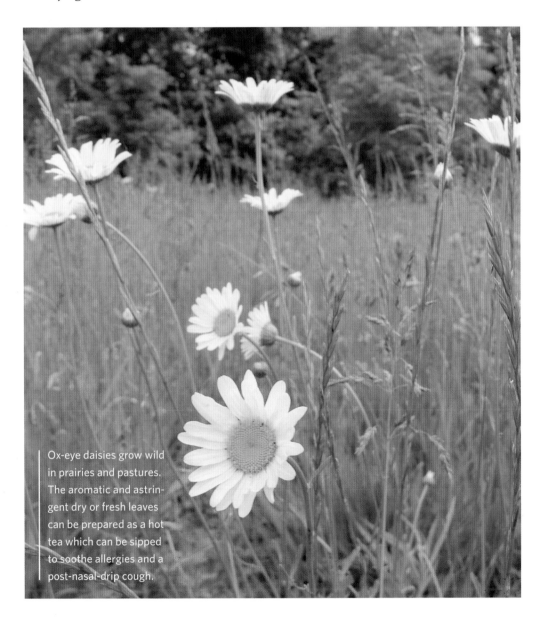

Ox-eye daisies grow wild in prairies and pastures. The aromatic and astringent dry or fresh leaves can be prepared as a hot tea which can be sipped to soothe allergies and a post-nasal-drip cough.

How to Identify

Ox-eye daisy is a clumping perennial. In early spring, emerging from a basal rosette, long and aromatic leaves are lance-shaped, toothed to lobed, sometimes shiny, hairy or smooth, and arranged alternately along the stem. The plant sends up flower stalks in June around the summer solstice and blossoms continue throughout the summer. Each flower is 1 to 1½ inches in diameter, with 20 white ray florets surrounding a yellow center disc.

Where, When, and How to Wildcraft

Look for ox-eye daisies in areas with damp soils in meadows, pastures, fields, and in planted gardens in full or partial sun. It spreads readily and is sometimes considered a noxious weed, especially when it grows in crop fields and pastures.

Gather the small, tender basal rosette leaves in the spring. They have a carroty odor. Plants become dry and rough later on in the season, particularly after the plant has gone to flower.

Pick the flower heads while in full bloom. Use them fresh or preserve them by drying the entire flower blossom on a screen. Store dried flowers in an airtight container to preserve freshness.

Medicinal Uses

Use ox-eye daisies as a first aid wound care remedy. Prepare the leaves and flowers as a topical wash to help astringe wet and weepy wounds, including rashes caused by poison ivy. Blend it with plants such as echinacea and plantain to help clear infections.

Prepare the aromatic and astringent leaves dry or fresh as a hot tea to soothe allergies and tickling coughs, and to dry a leaky, drippy, runny nose caused by early summer hay fever. Blend it with other drying aromatics such as ground ivy to help dry a runny nose and open sinuses.

Future Harvests

Ox-eye daisy is a common wildflower. Propagate plants using seeds or transplants from the original colony of plants.

HERBAL PREPARATIONS

Ox-eye daisy tea
Decoction
Drink ¼ cup as needed, or use as a topical wash.

Mitchella repens

PARTS USED leaves, stems

Partridge berry is a diminutive perennial plant and an astringent herb that helps tone and tighten prolapsed tissues.

How to Identify

Partridge berry is a low-growing plant, with 6- to 8-inch branches that creep along the forest floor. Its soft, hairless, round leaves are evergreen and ¾ inch in diameter; they grow in an opposite arrangement along the trailing stems.

Where they contact the soil, the stems form roots. Plants may grow into large colonies. In early spring, a joined pair of white, fragrant, funnel-shaped flowers emerge, which develop a single, red, terminal berry with two darker red spots on its surface. The berry is tasteless but is consumed by birds and other animals.

Unlike wintergreen leaves, which are also small, shiny, and evergreen, the leaves of partridge berry are relatively odorless but astringent in taste.

Where, When, and How to Wildcraft

Partridge berry grows in large stands as an abundant ground cover in mixed hardwood or coniferous forests, in dappled sunlight to deep shade. It winds around the bases of trees such as maples, hemlocks, and other conifers.

Collect the delicate leaves and stems across the season, taking care not to disturb the rootlets in the soil. Prepare the leaves and stems fresh as a tea or tincture or dry them for later use.

The tiny berries of the partridge berry provide bright dots of color on the forest floor in fall and winter. As a tea or tincture, the leaves can be combined with herbs like raspberry leaf to restore tone and strengthen weakened and prolapsed tissues.

Medicinal Uses

Partridge berry is markedly astringent. It is commonly used

to help tighten and tone tissues of both the female and male reproductive systems—namely, the uterus and prostate, respectively. In a tea, combine partridge berry with raspberry leaf for protocols to restore tone and strengthen weakened and prolapsed tissues.

Future Harvests

Partridge berry is commonly distributed throughout forests of the Midwest, but habitat loss is a concern for the sustainability of the plant. Harvest with care to avoid disturbing the rootlets. It is difficult to grow from seed but can be transplanted by cuttings to help start new stands in the woods or in the garden.

HERBAL PREPARATIONS

Partridge berry tea
Decoction
Drink ¼ cup as needed, or use topically as a wash.

pedicularis

Pedicularis canadensis
elephant head, lousewort, wood betony
PARTS USED flowers, leaves

*Pedicularis is a showy woodland plant that is useful as a relaxant herb
for muscle tension, and it helps relieve neck and back pain.*

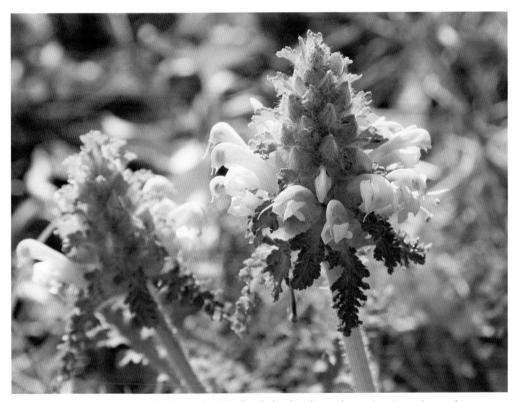

Pedicularis is a useful relaxant herb, particularly for skeletal and muscle tension. It can be used as a massage oil for spasming muscles and neck tension, as well as a tea or tincture.

How to Identify

Pedicularis is a low-growing perennial that starts as a basal rosette in spring. Leaves grow to 6 inches long and 2 inches wide; they are hairy, thick, and lance-shaped, with fernlike lobes.

In late spring, a flowering stalk covered with tiny hairs produces 1-inch-wide, slightly fragrant, two-lipped, tubular flowers. The upper lip curves downward (like an elephant's trunk) and functions as a protective hood, and the lower lip serves as a landing pad for insects. The flowers are usually yellow but can sometimes be brownish red.

Where, When, and How to Wildcraft

You'll find pedicularis in the dappled sun of open woodlands, prairies, and thickets, growing in well-drained, moist soils. Its showy blooms emerge in early spring, which is a good time to gather its flowers and leaves. Carefully gather these aerial parts by hand and use them fresh or dry them for later use.

Medicinal Uses

Use pedicularis as a tea or tincture, or infuse it in oil for massage, to relieve muscle spasms and neck tension. For a massage oil blend, mix pedicularis with other musculoskeletal herbs such as crampbark, goldenrod, and mullein root to ease back tension. Add St. John's wort if sharp, shooting nerve pain is present. These combinations can also be prepared as a tincture taken internally or used topically as a liniment.

Future Harvests

Pedicularis is limited in distribution; gather only the aerial parts to ensure future harvests.

 Cautions, Concerns, and Considerations

Pedicularis is a parasitic plant and may take up the toxins released by neighboring plant foliage. Make sure that you harvest in areas where pedicularis is not growing alongside poisonous plants, such as poison hemlock.

HERBAL PREPARATIONS

Pedicularis tea
Decoction
Drink ¼ cup as needed.

Pedicularis tincture
1 part fresh flowers and leaves, chopped
2 parts menstruum (50 percent alcohol, 50 percent distilled water)
Take 10–15 drops as needed.

Pedicularis-infused oil
1 part fresh flowers and leaves, chopped
2 parts oil
Use for massage.

---

pennycress

Thlaspi arvense
field pennycress
PARTS USED seeds

Pennycress seeds can be used similarly to mustard seeds in an herbal plaster to soothe muscle pain and ease damp and stagnant lung congestion.

How to Identify
A member of the mustard family (Brassicaceae), pennycress is an abundant-growing biennial plant (or weed) that emerges as a 6-inch-wide basal rosette in its first year. In the second year, its branching stems grow erect, to 24 inches in height. Oblong leaves are slightly lobed and grow in an alternate arrangement on the central stem. The lower leaves have short petioles or are sessile (without petioles), while the middle to upper leaves clasp the stem. Leaves produce a garlic smell when crushed.

Also in the plant's second year, racemes of tiny white flowers emerge in late spring and last through midsummer. Each flower is replaced by a heart-shaped seedpod up to ½ inch long and across. Seedpods produce small, aromatic, brownish black seeds that are useful as a medicinal or culinary spice.

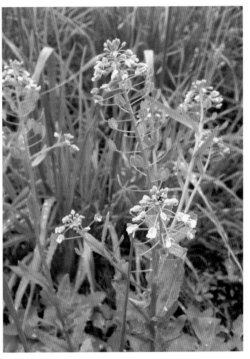

Pennycress is a wild weed, abundant in open fields and empty lots with rocky, disturbed soil. Collect the heart-shaped seedpods of the second-year plants in midsummer.

Where, When, and How to Wildcraft
Look for pennycress in open fields and empty lots, where it grows in rocky, disturbed soil. Collect the heart-shaped seedpods of second-year plants in midsummer by clipping the entire stem into a brown paper bag to avoid losing seeds. To preserve the seeds, winnow the papery husks from the seeds and store the huskless seeds in an airtight container.

Medicinal Uses
Pennycress seeds are used in a plaster, a poultice, or paste created with powdered seeds that can be applied over the skin to warm muscle tissues and relieve aches and pains. This works especially well on lower back rheumatic pain.

Pennycress plasters also increase circulation and ease tissue congestion. For stagnant lung congestion, apply the plaster to the chest or the back to help stimulate a productive cough.

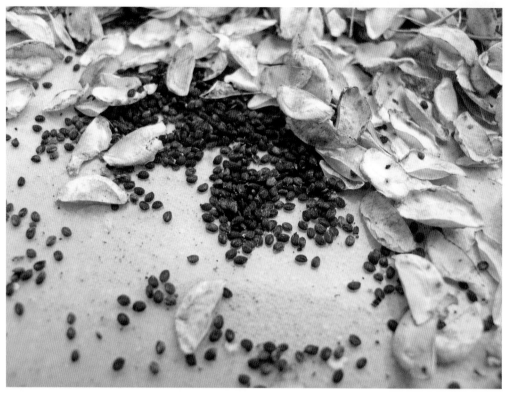

Spicy, aromatic, and stimulating, pennycress seeds are prepared and applied as a topical plaster to increase circulation and ease stagnant respiratory or musculo-skeletal congestion.

Future Harvests

Like other plants in the mustard family, pennycress is self-sowing and reproduces rapidly. It qualifies as an invasive weed in some areas. Harvesting pennycress from the wild will not impact future harvests.

 ## Cautions, Concerns, and Considerations

Do not apply the pennycress seed plaster directly to the skin; it can cause severe irritation.

HERBAL PREPARATIONS

Pennycress seed plaster
4 tablespoons seeds, ground
8 tablespoons wheat flour
1 pinch ground cayenne
1 pinch ginger
Grind the seeds using a mortar and pestle. Combine the seed powder and wheat flour. Add hot water to thicken the mixture to a paste. Add a pinch of ground cayenne and ginger to increase the stimulating effects (don't get this in your eyes).

To apply the plaster, place a warm, damp cloth over the skin and apply the warm paste in a thin layer on the cloth—applying the paste directly to the skin can cause severe irritation.

peppermint

Mentha ×piperita

PARTS USED flowers, leaves, stems

Peppermint is an herbalist's best friend. This stimulating aromatic is useful for a wide variety of maladies, from clearing a headache, to soothing a tummy, to encouraging a productive fever. It is a must for every herbalist's apothecary.

How to Identify
Peppermint is a creeping perennial that grows to 24 inches tall. Leaves are lance-shaped, toothed, and strongly aromatic, arranged oppositely on durable square stems that range in color from green, to red, to brown. Peppermint produces small white to pale-purple flower heads in early summer, after which the plant dries significantly and begins to die back.

Where, When, and How to Wildcraft
Look for this widely growing plant in moist, well-drained soil along stream banks and in woodlands in partial sun. Harvest leaves when they are most tender and aromatic in midspring, before flowering, for the best flavor—although flowers, leaves, and stems can be gathered at any time throughout the growing season. Use your nose and taste buds to determine the flavor and quality.

Plants grow rougher and spicier as the weather warms and before they flower, after which they become significantly drier. The tender leaves will return in the late fall when the weather cools.

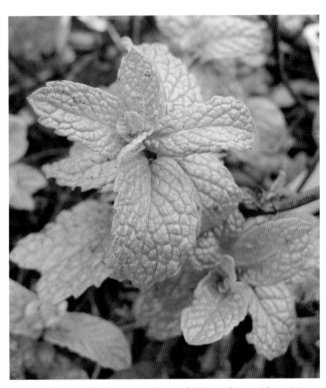

This useful, stimulating aromatic can help soothe a wide variety of maladies including clearing a headache, soothing a tummy, or helping stimulate a productive fever.

After gathering full stems of peppermint, bundle and hang them to dry for tea, or use the plant fresh. One or two armful-sized bundles can make enough tea for a family of four for winter's use. The fresh herb stores for up to a week when wrapped in a moist tea towel in the refrigerator, but for maximum aroma, process the plant immediately upon harvesting.

Medicinal Uses

Peppermint is a stimulating aromatic that is useful in clearing brain fog and lifting spirits in a simple cup of tea. Drink refreshing iced peppermint tea or a peppermint *agua fresca* (a fresh herb–water blend) to cool off on a warm day.

The hot tea is relaxant and soothing, and peppermint's aroma can help shoo away winter malaise or lull you to sleep at the end of the day. It can also soothe an upset stomach caused by the flu or by a case of butterflies and nerves.

For colds and flus, use peppermint to help support a productive fever. When blended with elderflower and yarrow, it makes an excellent cold and flu tea that can help boost the body's peripheral immune system to ward off the illness.

Peppermint is also a must for that perfect summertime classic: the mojito. One mojito can be medicinal. Two mojitos? Well, then it's a party. Three? Make peppermint tea the next morning.

Future Harvests

Peppermint spreads voraciously by underground runners, and gathering its long stalks will do little to affect the plant's future growth and harvest.

HERBAL PREPARATIONS

Peppermint tea
Infusion
Drink ½ cup as needed.

Peppermint tincture
1 part fresh flowers, leaves, and stems, chopped
2 parts menstruum (50 percent alcohol, 50 percent distilled water)
or
1 part dry flowers, leaves, and stems, chopped
4 parts menstruum (50 percent alcohol, 50 percent distilled water)
Take 15–20 drops as needed.

pine

Pinus species
PARTS USED bark, needles, resin

Use aromatic pine needles and resins to create teas and salves to soothe a sore throat or care for wounds. Pine salve can also help prevent chafing and windburn.

How to Identify
Pines are conifers that can grow up to 250 feet tall when mature. With most species, pine bark is gray, thick, and scaly, but some bark is smooth and green-gray in color. Branches grow spirally around the trunk. Soft, long, and flexible needles cluster in groups of two to five, depending on the species. Pines produce cones that mature after about two years and then fall to the ground. Female cones contain seeds that are eaten and dispersed by animals.

Where, When, and How to Wildcraft
Pines are the most common conifers in the world, and you'll find them growing in a variety of locations, from sandy soils along lakes, to forested areas, to old farmsteads and active urban landscapes. Most pines prefer acidic soils. Wild pines grow in large stands.

Collect needles by hand at any time; they are most tender and aromatic in the spring, which is also the best time to collect bark and resin. To gather the bark, trim it from small twigs and branches to use in teas or tinctures. Scrape the resin from the sides of the tree to use for salve. Store it in a sealed container.

Medicinal Uses
Use pine needles to make an aromatic tea. Not only are they rich in vitamin C, but pine needle aromatics are extremely useful in

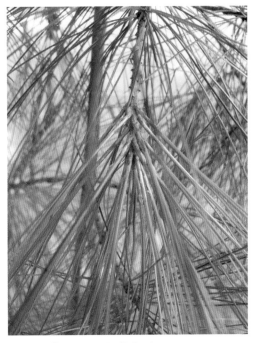

Pine needles grow spirally in clumps.

clearing stuffy sinus congestion from winter colds. To make tea, add boiling water and needles to a teapot, cover, and let steep for 3 to 5 minutes. Sweeten the needle tea with honey, and inhale the fragrance as you sip. A steaming pot of needles also makes an excellent steam inhalation to clear sinus congestion, used similarly to a eucalyptus steam.

Pine is also markedly resinous, and the young bark, needles, and resins can be extracted in high-proof alcohol to create a tincture to use for wound care and sore

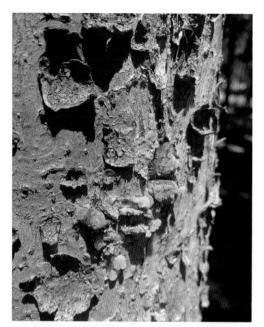

Pine resin is a useful first aid remedy that can be applied from the tree as a field bandage to cover scrapes and cuts, as well as used in the mouth to cover cankerous sores.

throats. Pine resin can also be used in the mouth to cover cankerous sores, or use it directly from the tree as a sticky field bandage to cover scrapes and cuts. Pine resin can be infused into olive oil to create a divine aromatic massage oil or to prepare as a salve by mixing with beeswax.

Future Harvests

Harvest bark, needles, and resin in a sustainable manner by gathering them from fallen branches after a windstorm. Transplant pine seedlings into areas with acidic soils. Advocacy for habitat protection and restoration will help increase the distribution of white pine across the Midwest.

HERBAL PREPARATIONS

Pine needle tea
Infusion
Drink ½ cup as needed, or use the steaming pot for steam inhalation.

Pine tincture
1 part fresh bark, needles, and resin, chopped
2 parts menstruum (95 percent alcohol, 5 percent distilled water)
Take 10–15 drops as needed.

Pine resin–infused oil
1 part resin
2 parts olive oil
Use for massage.

pipsissewa

Chimaphila umbellata

PARTS USED leaves

Pipsissewa is an astringent and stimulating plant medicine that is used to restore tone to the urinary tract and tissues.

How to Identify

Pipsissewa is a flowering woodland plant that grows 4–14 inches tall. Bright evergreen leaves are toothed and ovate with deep veins. Leaves grow in whorls arranged in opposite pairs along the stem. In summer, a 4-inch flower stalk bears branched umbels of pinkish white flowers.

Where, When, and How to Wildcraft

Look for pipsissewa in the acidic soils beneath conifers in the dappled shade of woodlands. Gather the evergreen leaves year-round. Carefully gather one or two leaves per plant to avoid disrupting the plant's ability to photosynthesize. Prepare them fresh into medicine or dry them for later use.

Medicinal Uses

Pipsissewa can help restore tone to urinary tissues when prepared as a tea or tincture. This medicinal plant is especially helpful in protocols that address chronic urinary tract infections with damp, prolapsed urinary tissues.

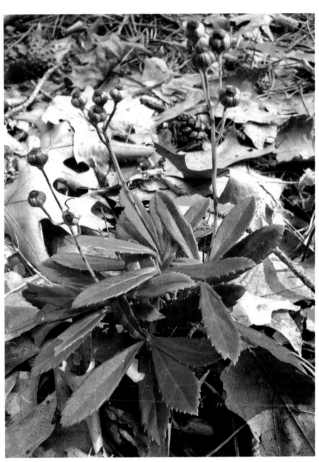

Pipsissewa grows in dappled shade. It is a stimulating and astringent plant that can help restore tone to urinary tissues when prepared as a tea or tincture.

Integrate other herbs with affinities to the urinary tract into an herbal protocol along with pipsissewa, such as cranberry, corn silk, echinacea, and uva-ursi. Use wild yam with pipsissewa to relieve painful spasms in the urinary tract and kidney area.

Future Harvests

Pipsissewa is on the watch list by herbalists because of overharvesting and loss of habitat. Gather it mindfully.

Cautions, Concerns, and Considerations

Pipsissewa is notably stimulating and should not be used in long-term treatment.

HERBAL PREPARATIONS

Pipsissewa tea
Decoction
Drink ¼ cup as needed.

Pipsissewa tincture
1 part fresh or dry leaves, chopped
2 parts menstruum (50 percent alcohol, 50 percent distilled water)
Take 10–15 drops as needed.

plantain

Plantago species
PARTS USED leaves, seeds

The wild and weedy plantain is a primary tissue-healer in the herbal apothecary. It is useful in wound care and in promoting internal healing of ulcerous tissues.

How to Identify

Plantain grows as a basal rosette of broad or narrow leaves. The broadleaf plantain's smooth, parallel-veined foliage grows up to 6 inches long and 4 inches wide. The leaf stems are fibrous and can have a red tinge at the base. The foliage of the narrow-leaved plantain is slightly more dry and hairy, with leaves 6–8 inches long that are lance-shaped and pointed.

Both types produce long flower stalks in midsummer, covered with small white blossoms that give way to small, edible seeds. The husk (the outer covering of the seed) is a great source of dietary fiber and is commonly sold in health food stores as psyllium husks.

Where, When, and How to Wildcraft

Look for plantain growing anywhere people live: in yards and parks, in sidewalk cracks, and along the trail. Make a note not to gather plantain where dogs may stop along the trail.

The fresh, clean leaves of plantain are best gathered in spring while they are the most vibrant and tender, but you can harvest them across the season. Look for the dry brown seeds in late summer, winnow them from the flower stalk, and store them in an airtight container.

Medicinal Uses

Plantain is best known for its ability to support wound healing. It helps moderate tissue

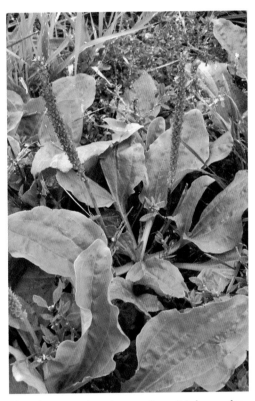

Plantain grows almost everywhere. It is known for its abilities to support wound healing while helping to prevent infection from setting in.

healing while working to prevent septic infection. Prepare plantain as a topical wash for cleaning wounds (especially spider bites and poison ivy), as a tincture for internal use or diluted for a topical wash, or as a salve for a healing topical balm. Plantain pairs well with chickweed, goldenrod, St. John's wort, and yarrow in a healing salve.

Plantain tea soothes internal, inflamed intestinal conditions as part of herbal protocols that help heal ulcers and alleviate inflammatory bowel issues. It works well in combination with marshmallow root.

Psyllium seeds are useful as binder ingredients in gluten-free baking, and because of their mucilaginous, expansive qualities, they are good for anyone who wants to add healing fiber to their diet.

Future Harvests

Plantain reseeds easily and grows ubiquitously, so you can harvest it without impacting the sustainability of the plant.

HERBAL PREPARATIONS

Plantain tea
Decoction
Drink ½ cup as needed, or use topically as a wound wash.

Plantain tincture
1 part fresh leaves, chopped
2 parts menstruum (50 percent alcohol, 50 percent distilled water)
Take 10–15 drops as needed.

Plantain-infused oil
1 part fresh leaves, chopped
2 parts oil
Use for massage.

poke

Phytolacca americana
American pokeweed, pokeweed
PARTS USED roots

Poke root has long been used in plant medicine particularly in the southeastern US. It is useful as a lymphatic herb to support the immune system in times of septic infection.

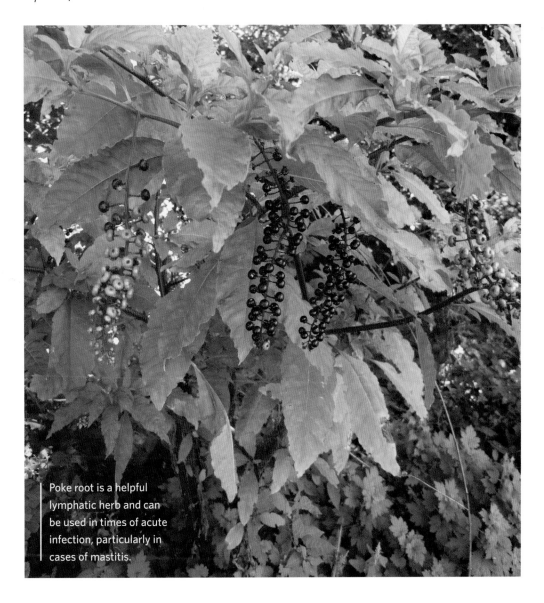

Poke root is a helpful lymphatic herb and can be used in times of acute infection, particularly in cases of mastitis.

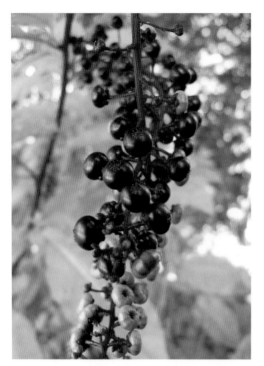

Poke's small whitish-green flower clusters bloom in early summer and develop drooping clusters of beautiful dark purple berries in late summer. The stalk and the leaf stems become magenta-colored as the season progresses.

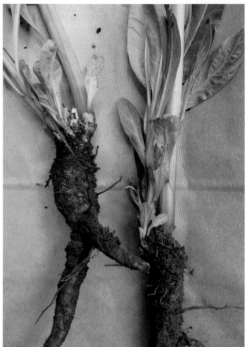

Poke root helps clear plugged mammary ducts and relieves the systemic infection of mastitis which can quickly ensue if not addressed immediately. Poke root is best combined as a tincture in equal parts with echinacea and red root (ceanothus).

How to Identify

Growing 6–8 feet tall, poke is an herbaceous perennial, with purplish tubular stalks that may be striped in bright pink. Its leaves are a vibrant green with wavy margins and a smooth and waxy texture, arranged alternately on the stem.

The perennial plant pushes up through the ground in midspring, flowers in early summer, and develops berries in late July and into August. Small white-green flower clusters bloom in early summer and develop into drooping clusters of dark purple berries in late summer. The stalks and leaf stems turn magenta as the season progresses. Poke roots are branching, white, and fleshy.

Where, When, and How to Wildcraft

Poke thrives in a wide range of poor soils, from heavy clay to acidic, sandy soils. It grows in disturbed ground and in waste places alongside burdock and various evergreens. Using a shovel, dig the roots at any time. Dry them or prepare them fresh in an oil infusion or tincture.

Medicinal Uses

Poke is a common medicinal herb used frequently in the southeastern United States. It is a helpful lymphatic herb in times of acute infection—particularly for mastitis, a terribly uncomfortable and painful ailment of nursing mothers caused by inflamed, plugged milk ducts. Poke root helps clear the plugged duct and relieves the systemic infection that can quickly ensue if mastitis is not addressed immediately.

Poke root is best combined as a tincture in equal parts with ceanothus and echinacea, which can be used topically or internally. Concurrently, apply poke root oil liberally to the breast area and cover with a hot, damp cloth to help stimulate the clearing of the milk duct.

Future Harvests

Poke is a common wild plant. Harvesting its roots will disturb the plant but will not impact its abundance throughout the Midwest.

 ### Cautions, Concerns, and Considerations

This plant is recommended for use only by seasoned herbalists. Some conventional literature notes that poke berries and roots are poisonous in any amount; however, these plant parts are widely used by experienced herbalists in Southern folk medicine. If the berries are consumed and there is concern about poisoning, contact poison control and consume plain yogurt to stabilize the stomach. Watch for vomiting or other signs of poisoning. Although the debate against poke's use is widely unsubstantiated, if in doubt choose to work with another herb.

HERBAL PREPARATIONS

Poke root tincture
1 part fresh roots, chopped
2 parts menstruum (50 percent alcohol, 50 percent distilled water)
Take 10–15 drops as needed.

Poke root–infused oil
1 part fresh roots, chopped
2 parts oil
Use for massage.

prickly ash

Zanthoxylum americanum
toothache tree
PARTS USED bark

Prickly ash is sometimes known as the toothache tree because its bark is used as a numbing agent for dental pain.

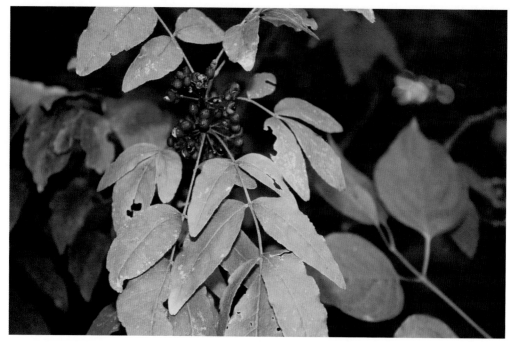

Gather the bark in early spring from twigs and branches. It can be used fresh or dried.

How to Identify

Prickly ash is an understory shrub that is typically 5 to 8 feet tall, but it can sometimes grow to 20 feet in height. Plants form tight thickets that are difficult to penetrate because of the stout, paired, half-inch–long spines that grow at nodes along the stems and branches. Its alternate, dark green leaves are pinnately compound, with 5–13 leaflets.

Prickly ash shrubs can be misidentified as black locust saplings because both have thorns and compound leaves. Black locust

leaflets are elliptical, however, while prickly ash leaflets taper to a point. Black locust produces white racemes of fragrant flowers in early summer, while prickly ash flowers are produced in small axillary clusters in the spring before the plant leafs out; they are about ⅛ inch long and green to yellow-green in color.

Prickly ash fruit is a red, roundish, warty pod that grows in dense clusters close to the twig. It splits open from late July to mid-September to reveal a single glossy, black seed. The fruit has a strong citrus fragrance. Bite into it, however, and you will find it bitter and numbing.

Where, When and How to Wildcraft

Look for prickly ash growing along the edges of woodlands, in open fields, along bluffs, and in disturbed soils. Gather the bark in early spring from twigs and branches. Use it fresh or dry it for later use.

Medicinal Uses

Create a bark tincture and dilute it in water to use as a dental rinse to numb tender gum areas. Generally, most acute dental issues are accompanied by inflammation, and this numbing plant medicine works well with a mouth rinse of astringent plantain and oak bark to help tighten and tone the dental tissues.

Future Harvests

Prickly ash reproduces abundantly, and the bark and berries can be gathered without impacting future harvests. In fact, harvesting the plant will help keep it from spreading across disturbed soils.

HERBAL PREPARATIONS

Prickly ash tincture
1 part fresh bark, chopped
2 parts menstruum (95 percent alcohol,
  5 percent distilled water)
Take 15–20 drops as needed; add to water for dental rinse.

prickly pear

Opuntia species
PARTS USED fruit, pads

Similar to aloe, prickly pear juice is cooling and soothing to the touch and can be used for burns and skin healing.

How to Identify
Prickly pear is a perennial cactus that grows to about 24 inches tall in the Midwest. Its flat, blue-green, rounded pads (cladodes) are 2–8 inches long, 1½ to 5 inches across, and ½ inch to 1¼ inches thick. Large spines ½ inch to 4 inches long grow from pores (areoles) on the pads and fruits (tunas), along with tiny, hairy spines (glochids) that are also scattered across each pad.

Flowers bloom in early summer and produce 1- to 2-inch succulent, reddish brown fruit that can be harvested through the fall. Fruit may taste sour, bland, or sweet. The entire plant shrivels and dries in late fall, after the first frosts.

Where, When, and How to Wildcraft
Prickly pear grows in colonies, spreading across disturbed sandy and rocky soils, in south-facing, sunny locations. It is commonly cultivated as a landscape plant.

Harvest the pads across the growing season, choosing those that are green and firm. Gather the fruits when they are brightly colored and succulent, before the plant begins to die back in the late fall.

In the kitchen, wear gloves as you work with the pads and fruits. To remove the glochids, hold the pad or fruit with tongs over an open flame to burn off the spines. After they are burned off, you can peel, chop, or puree the fruit and pads.

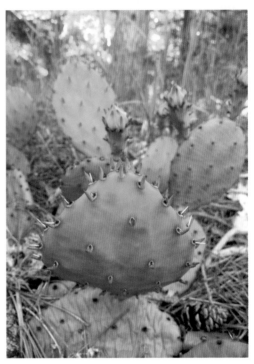

The inner core of prickly pear has a cooling and astringent action similar to that of aloe and can be used for skin healing.

Medicinal Uses
Prickly pear pads and fruit possess cooling and astringent actions that are helpful for skin healing for burn relief, including sunburn.

Future Harvests
Prickly pear can be propagated by cuttings and grows easily in disturbed, rocky, and sandy soils. Plant it in a south-facing, sunny area for the most prolific growth.

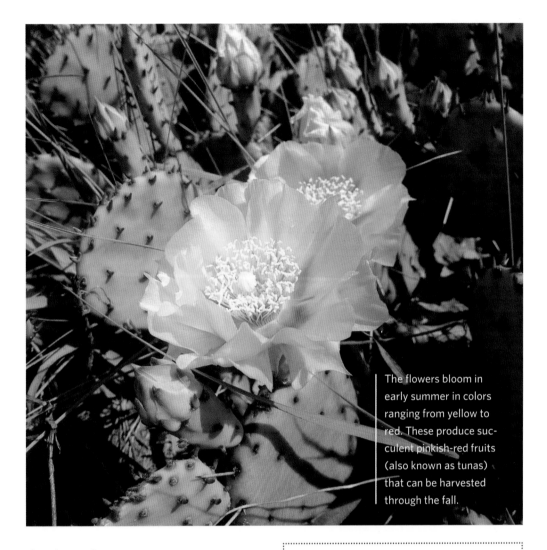

The flowers bloom in early summer in colors ranging from yellow to red. These produce succulent pinkish-red fruits (also known as tunas) that can be harvested through the fall.

Cautions, Concerns, and Considerations

Both pads and fruit are covered in large and tiny spines. Although the large spines are somewhat avoidable, the glochids are pesky buggers that can get into your skin and feel like a fiberglass rash. The glochids will embed into fabric, too, so do your gathering wearing leather gloves and harvest the pads and fruit directly into a paper bag (the tiny spines could never be removed from a fabric harvest bag, ruining it for reuse) or a solid-surface bowl.

HERBAL PREPARATIONS

Prickly pear healing balm

Remove the glochids and spines from a pad or fruit and peel.

Apply the peeled material topically to burned skin, and cover the area with a cool, damp cloth.

Rubus species
red raspberry (*R. idaeus*), black raspberry (*R. occidentalis*)
PARTS USED fruit, leaves, roots

Prepare raspberry leaves as a mineral-dense tea or broth to help astringe wet and weepy wounds (such as a poison ivy rash). Raspberry fruit is also a yummy trail snack for your medicine-wildcrafting adventures.

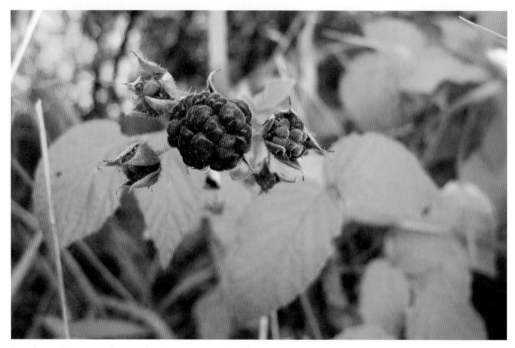

Raspberry leaves are known for their vitamin C and are rich mineral content. The leaves are high in calcium, potassium, iron, zinc, and phosphorus as well as vitamins A, C, E, and B.

How to Identify

Thorny canes of red and black raspberries grow 7–10 feet tall in large thickets. Pinnately compound leaves have three to five toothed leaflets and grow alternately on the stem; they are primarily green with silvery undersides. Both species produce white flowers in late spring. Black raspberries ripen in midsummer, and red raspberries ripen in late summer to early fall.

Where, When, and How to Wildcraft

You'll find this native woodlander at the edges of the woods, or along trails, hedgerows, and ditches.

Gather the leaves in the early spring before the plant begins to develop flowers, usually in early June. The leaves can also be gathered again in the late fall after the plant is done fruiting. If you are thinning a stand of raspberry canes, the entire cane can be

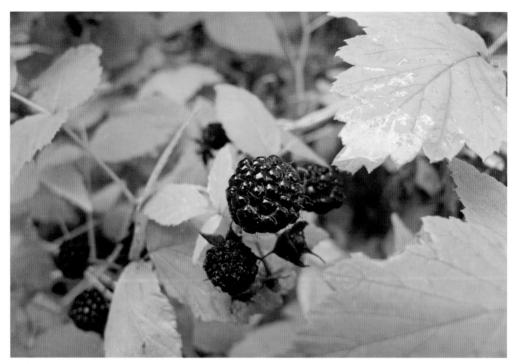
The leaves of black raspberry can be used similarly as the red.

pruned and stripped of its leaves to use fresh or to dry on a screen.

Pick the ripe fruits of black raspberry in early July and red raspberry in August to early September. Use the fruit right away or freeze it. Gather the berries in the summer sun when the high amounts of sugar in the fruit make it sweeter.

You can dig the roots at any time, though this may be easiest to do when you are thinning the canes, using a shovel and clippers. The roots are quite spindly, so a considerable amount of them are needed for preservation. Use them fresh or chop and dry them for later use.

Medicinal Uses
Raspberry leaves are high in calcium, iron, phosphorus, potassium, and zinc, as well as vitamins A, B complex, C, and E. For a mineral-dense tea, extract these nutrients by preparing a long decoction. Boil the leaves for 20 minutes and enjoy them in a strong tea, hot or iced. Raspberry leaves mix well in tea with nettle, oatstraw, and red clover for a mineral-rich drink. If the drink is too earthy in taste, add ice to mellow the flavor. Add aromatics such as spicebush or the barks of aspen, birch, or tulip poplar to spice up the beverage.

Raspberry leaf tea is astringent and can help tighten and tone prolapsed tissues. This tea is often recommended for women to help astringe and tone uterine tissues during childbearing years, specifically during pregnancy and postpartum. Because of its mineral density, it is also a helpful medicine to incorporate into herbal therapies to support hormone balance.

This beverage isn't only for women—it can also be added to protocols for men who need an astringent medicine to support healthy and toned prostate tissues. Consider pairing it with partridge berry for this use.

In the kitchen, add foraged mushrooms such as maitake, reishi, and turkey tail to raspberry leaf tea to create a delicious, nutrient-dense vegan broth base for soups and stews. Raspberry root tea is a traditional remedy for diarrhea. This astringent brew can be blended with cocoa or chai to help settle and dry up the condition and soothe the stomach and digestive tract. Add honey to sweeten.

Future Harvests

Raspberries are easily propagated by cuttings or by transplanting the canes. They spread quickly and are tolerant of a lazy gardener. You can attach the canes to a trellis or let them grow untouched along a woodland edge as part of a permaculture landscape plan. Because raspberry is a voracious perennial spreader, gathering its leaves and fruits will have a minimal impact on future harvests.

HERBAL PREPARATIONS

Raspberry leaf tea
Decoction
Drink 1 cup per day as needed, or use topically as a wound wash.

Raspberry root tea
Decoction
Drink ¼ cup as needed.

Raspberry vinegar shrub
1 part fresh berries and leaves, crushed
2 parts raw apple cider vinegar
Take 2–3 tablespoons per day.

red clover

Trifolium pratense
PARTS USED flowers, leaves

Red clover, with its abundance of minerals, is an important functional food that supports tissue health.

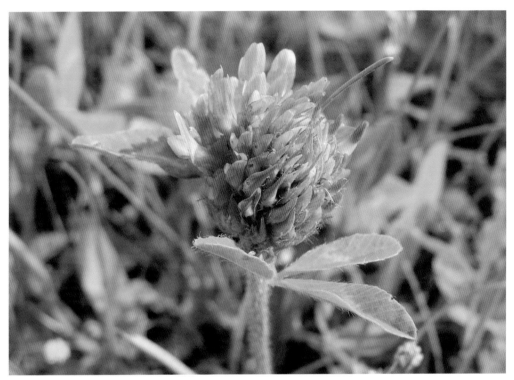

Red clover extraction mixes well with nettle, oat straw, horsetail, or raspberry to make a nutrient-dense beverage which can be enjoyed as an iced or room-temperature tea.

How to Identify

This low-spreading perennial grows to 12 inches tall. Leaves, which alternate along the stem, are trifoliate (with three leaflets), with a pale chevron shape on the outer part of each leaf. The stem of red clover is hairy. Flowers blossom in June, with a showy pink-purple head comprising many small, nectar-filled, tubular florets, which attract a variety of pollinators.

Where, When, and How to Wildcraft

Look for red clover growing abundantly in sunny, open spaces in moist or dry soils. Red clover begins to bloom in June, near the solstice, and remains in bloom throughout the summer. Gather the blossoms and top greens by hand or with scissors on a dry, sunny day. Choose only the flowers and leaves that are vibrant and free of brown withering. Do not gather blossoms that are damp or wet because they will wilt or could mold before drying. Use the blossoms fresh or dry them on screens for later use.

Medicinal Uses

With its abundance of minerals, red clover is an important functional food for supporting tissue health. Extract fresh or dry plant material in a long decoction in hot water or boil for 20 minutes. Red clover mixes well with horsetail, nettle, oatstraw, or raspberry to make a nutrient-dense tea to enjoy iced or at room temperature.

Future Harvests

Red clover is an abundant wild plant. A perennial, it returns after being gathered or even mowed. Gathering the blossoms and leaves will not affect future harvests.

Cautions, Concerns, and Considerations

Although there has been some debate regarding clover's possible effects on hormone balance, traditional use suggests it is safe for consumption. Because red clover draws a significant amount of minerals from the soil, harvest only in areas that are free from pesticides, nitrate pollution, and heavy metal contamination.

HERBAL PREPARATIONS

Red clover tea
Decoction
Drink 1 cup as needed.

Ganoderma species

artist's conk (*G. applanatum*); hemlock varnish shelf (*G. tsugae*); ling chih, varnished conk (*G. lucidum*)

PARTS USED fruiting body

Reishi is a well-researched fungus that is popular in traditional Chinese medicine as an immune system stabilizer and nourishing tonic. Reishi is much needed for today's hectic and stressful lifestyle.

How to Identify

Mature reishi grows to 8–12 inches in diameter on hardwoods and conifers. The kidney-shaped conk has a shiny and smooth finish, in hues of deep reddish browns, usually with a whitish rim. The underside of the fruiting body has no gills and is dull white to brown with brown spores.

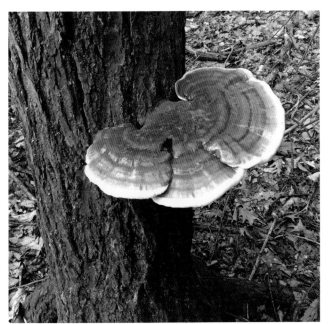

Reishi is most commonly used as a decoction as heat releases the nourishing polysaccharides. A reishi decoction can be blended with other nourishing herbs like burdock, nettle, and red clover.

Where, When, and How to Wildcraft

Reishi mushrooms are abundant in hardwood and coniferous forests throughout the Midwest, especially *G. tsugae*, which grows on the decaying wood of the hemlock tree.

Gather the fruiting body at any time of year by cutting it away from the tree with a sharp knife. Be sure to leave the base intact and attached to ensure that it will regrow.

To dry reishi, slice the mushroom and cure it in the sun. Traditional solar preparations maximize the release of vitamin D in the mushroom.

Medicinal Uses

Because of its increasing popularity, a lot of substandard reishi products are available commercially; wildcrafting it yourself makes sense and offers a wonderful addition to the home apothecary.

Reishi's polysaccharides help strengthen and stabilize the body's immune cells and immune response. Reishi is most important for convalescence or for individuals with

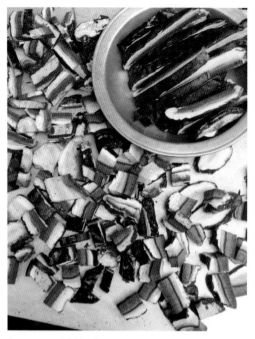

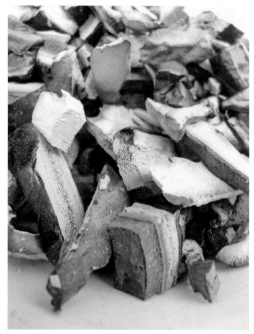

Sun-cure reishi in the summertime to maximize the release of vitamin D.

Dry reishi, ready for tea.

debility. It can help soothe nervous tension and stabilize a hyperactive immune response to outside variables such as cold, noise, and environmental allergies. It can also be used to help stabilize insulin levels.

A hot reishi decoction is the most common way to use the mushroom, because heat releases the nourishing polysaccharides. Blend reishi with other nourishing herbs such as burdock, nettle, and red clover. Or create a woodland chai tea by combining acorn hulls, burdock, reishi, and chai spices such as sassafras root, spicebush berries, and wild ginger; drink it daily to nourish the immune system in lieu of depleting beverages such as coffee.

Future Harvests

Reishi has an indeterminate growth habit, but a new fungus will grow only when the base remains attached to the tree. When you cut the fungus from the tree, be sure to leave the base intact and attached to preserve future harvests.

HERBAL PREPARATIONS

Reishi tea
Decoction
Drink ¼ cup per day.

Rosa species
wild rose
PARTS USED hips, leaves, petals

As a first aid remedy, wild rose petals and leaves are used as a topical wash to astringe burns and wet and weepy poison ivy rashes, and to dry up weepy, infected wounds.

How to Identify

Wild rose is a spreading shrub that grows to 5 feet tall. Its canes are thorny, with finely serrated, deep green, and shiny compound leaves that are arranged alternately. Rosebuds form in mid-June and open into five-petaled blossoms in a range of colors from white to dark pink. Flowers are 1–3 inches across, depending on the species.

After rose blossoms are pollinated by bees and other insects, fruit, or rose hips, form in late summer, ranging in diameter from ¼ inch to 1½ inches. Rose hips turn dark red when they are ripe, typically in mid- to late September.

Where, When, and How to Wildcraft

Look for wild roses in disturbed and rocky soils along woodland edges and near lakes and rivers. The heady perfume of the flowers rests on the summer breezes, guiding you to brambles filled with blossoms ready to be gathered by the basketful. Gather the flowers in early summer using pruners or scissors. Harvest on a dry, sunny day, because wet weather will diminish the aromatics. Gather blossoms from healthy plants only; roses are susceptible to mildew, blight, and aphids. Use the petals fresh or dry them flat on screens to use later.

Rose hips are best gathered in the fall when their flavors are most pronounced. On the larger rose hips, scoop out the seeds and the interior hairs around the seeds before drying them in a dehydrator or cooking them, to avoid possible throat irritation and stomach upset.

Gather the leaves at any time to prepare as

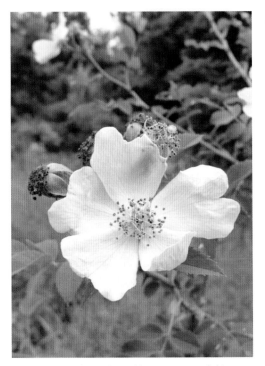

Astringent rose petals and leaves are useful in herbal medicine. As a topical wash they can astringe burns and wet, weepy rashes like poison ivy, and dry up weepy wounds that are filled with pus.

Herbal First Aid for Poison Ivy and Burns

Rose petals and calendula flowers are useful in a holistic vinegar infusion to soothe sunburns and kitchen burns, and to dry up a wet, weepy rash from poison ivy. Use this vinegar infusion in a spray bottle to mist sunburned skin or poison ivy rashes in hard-to-reach places.

Sunburn relief vinegar infusion

2 cups raw apple cider vinegar
4 tablespoons fresh or dry rose petals
2 tablespoons fresh or dry calendula flowers

1. Combine the vinegar and flowers in a quart jar and allow the mixture to sit for two weeks in the refrigerator.
2. Strain the mixture and store it in the refrigerator to use as needed for a wash or skin soak for burns. It will stay fresh for up to 6 months.

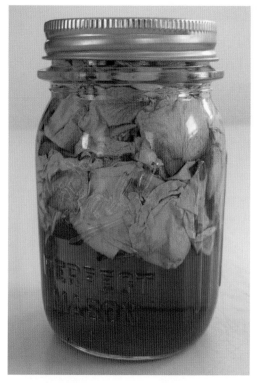

A vinegar infusion of rose petals makes a soothing burn relief spray.

an astringent topical wash. They can be used fresh or dried for later use.

Medicinal Uses

Rose petals and leaves are useful plant medicines for their astringent properties. Use them in a topical wash to astringe burns and wet and weepy rashes, and to dry up weepy wounds.

To create an exceptional burn relief spray, infuse rose petals in vinegar. The infusion soothes sunburns and culinary burns and should be on hand in every kitchen and in every first aid kit.

Energetically, roses are a heart tonic and can soothe heartache, depression, and sadness. The tea, tincture, elixir, and massage oils of the petals can be integrated into a self-care routine to ease a broken heart. Flower water made with rose petals lifts the spirits when spritzed onto the face or around a room.

Rose hips are high in vitamin C and can be collected and preserved in the fall, after a frost. Prepare them as a decoction to use in syrup, or dry them to add to tea blends.

Future Harvests

Wild rose is deemed a noxious weed in some areas. It is easily propagated by transplanting canes, and gathering its hips, leaves, and blossoms will not significantly impact future harvests.

HERBAL PREPARATIONS

Rose leaf tea
Infusion
Drink ½ cup as needed, or use topically as a wound wash.

Rose petal tea
Infusion
Drink 1 cup as needed.

Rose petal–infused vinegar
1 part fresh or dry rose petals
2 parts raw apple cider vinegar
Take 2–3 tablespoons as needed, or use as a topical wound wash.

Rose petal tincture
1 part fresh petals
2 parts menstruum (50 percent alcohol, 50 percent distilled water)
or
1 part dry petals
3 parts menstruum (50 percent alcohol, 50 percent distilled water)
Take 10–15 drops as needed.

Rose petal–infused oil
1 part fresh petals
2 parts oil
Use for massage.

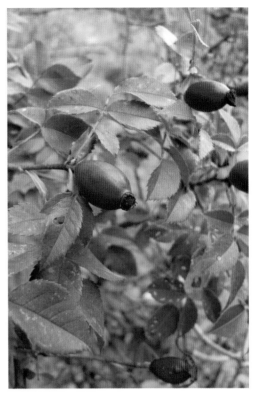

Rose hips are high in vitamin C and can be collected and preserved in the early fall; they are most sweet after a frost.

Russian sage

Perovskia atriplicifolia
PARTS USED flowers, leaves

A common ornamental flowering plant, Russian sage is a useful medicinal herb for soothing an upset stomach, treating a cold or flu, or washing a wound.

How to Identify
Russian sage is a perennial in the mint family that typically grows from 2 to 4 feet, with upright, square stems. Leaves are finely dissected, aromatic when crushed, and silvery in color. Throughout the summer, lavender-blue tubular flowers are arranged in panicles along the upper part of each stem.

Where, When, and How to Wildcraft
Common in landscaping as well as abandoned gardens, Russian sage can be gathered in abundance when the plant is in full bloom from late summer to early fall. Bundle entire branches and hang them to dry for later use, or strip the flowers and leaves to be processed fresh into medicinal preparations.

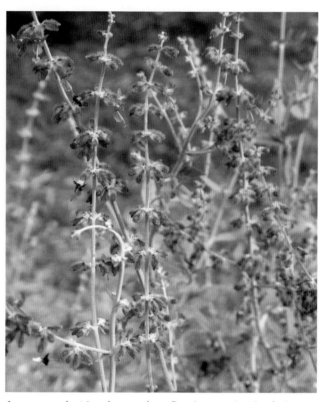

A common plant in urban gardens, Russian sage is stimulating and aromatic, its volatile oils useful for clearing sinuses in an inhalation steam or simply soothing a head cold.

Medicinal Uses
Although it is not a member of the genus *Salvia*, Russian sage shares many commonalities with white and culinary sage. Russian sage is stimulating and aromatic, and its volatile oils are useful for clearing sinuses or soothing a head cold with an inhalation steam.

To treat colds and flus, Russian sage blends well in a tea with elderflower, spotted bee balm, wild bergamot, and yarrow. It lends a unique flavor when infused in honey, and when the infusion is added to tea, it creates an aromatic and antimicrobial blend (and it's nice drizzled over local goat cheese).

Russian sage tea or tincture can help relieve a sinus or barometric-pressure headache and dispel gas and bloating that may follow overindulgence or a heavy meal. Its aromatics are also useful for soothing nervous anxiety and tension.

Prepare massage oil with Russian sage to stimulate circulation, especially during winter to help warm the body. Use dried Russian sage bundles for room smudging, or heat the dried sage in water to create steam to dispel negative energy or clear the room of stagnant air.

Future Harvests

Russian sage is a common landscape plant that grows throughout the Midwest. Gathering branches of this perennial for tea and other preparations will not significantly affect future harvests.

HERBAL PREPARATIONS

Russian sage tea
Infusion
Drink ½ cup as needed.

Russian sage tincture
1 part fresh flowers and leaves, chopped
2 parts menstruum (50 percent alcohol, 50 percent distilled water)
Take 15 drops as needed.

Russian sage–infused honey
1 part fresh flowers and leaves, chopped
3 parts raw, unpasteurized honey
Use as needed.

Russian sage–infused oil
1 part fresh flowers and leaves, chopped
2 parts oil
Use for massage.

Sassafras albidum
PARTS USED leaves, root bark

Sassafras is a delicious spicy and aromatic medicinal plant that is used to soothe sore throats, calm upset stomachs, and open the sinuses.

How to Identify

Sassafras is a slender deciduous tree that reaches 60 feet or more in optimum conditions. Its reddish-brown bark is deeply furrowed.

Yellow to greenish yellow flowers are produced in loose, drooping racemes up to 2 inches long in early spring, shortly before the leaves appear. Sassafras trees are dioecious, with either male or female flowers on separate trees. The female flowers have no sepals (the leaflike green structures at the bases of flowers). Oval blue-black fruit ripens in late summer.

Leaves are smooth-edged and soft and alternate along the stem. Some leaves are ovate with no lobe, others are mitten-shaped, and still others have three distinct lobes. The aromatic roots range in color from white to reddish brown. The entire plant is fragrant, with a scent similar to spicy root beer or fruit-flavored cereal.

Where, When, and How to Wildcraft

Sassafras thrives in partial sun in sandy, well-drained soil along trails and roadsides, fence lines, orchards, beach areas, and woodlands. Harvest the leaves at any time, though the young leaves early in the season are more tender, fragrant, and cooling. Dry leaves flat on a screen and store them in an airtight container.

Gather the roots from small saplings in the spring or fall. Peel the bark from

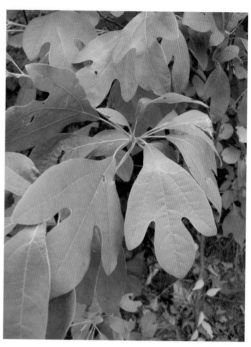

Try sassafras leaves in the heat of the summer sun for a sweet, cooling taste of the plant's aromatic flavor. Its mucilaginous leaves can be extracted into cool water with slippery elm to make a cool infusion that will soothe a sore throat or dry a cough.

the roots, and then wash, chop, and dry it completely. You can also gather the tree bark from small branches in the spring, but its aroma at this time isn't as pronounced or as pleasing as that of the root bark.

Medicinal Uses

Extract sassafras's mucilaginous leaves with slippery elm in cool water to make an

A Mitten Gal's Herbal Root Beer

While on a trail run through the dunes near my home, I realized that no other smell is more reminiscent of my West Michigan lakeshore upbringing than sassafras. That spicy root beer fragrance of the sassafras floats on the breeze in the dew of the morning or after a rain. It is one of those scents that truly defines my life.

You can make simple syrup with aromatic sassafras and other woodland herbs to create a batch of herbal root beer. Drink this beverage to soothe a tummy ache, or simply enjoy it as a refreshing cooler.

Herbal simple syrup

½ cup dry sassafras root bark, chopped
¼ cup dry burdock root, chopped
1 tablespoon dry hops, chopped
1 teaspoon dry whole juniper berries
10 wintergreen leaves, chopped
1 teaspoon dry ginger root, chopped
1 teaspoon spicebush berries (optional)
4 cups water
4 cups Michigan maple syrup

1. Add 1 part sassafras simple syrup mixture to 2 parts club soda and serve over ice or top with vanilla ice cream.
2. Sassafras simple syrup can be stored in the fridge for up to 3 weeks.

infusion that soothes a sore throat or a dry, barking cough. Add cherry bark to help relax the cough. Lemon balm, linden flowers, rose petals, and violet flowers and leaves all work well combined with sassafras leaves for a pleasant herbal infusion. Pulverize the dry leaves and mix them with honey, lavender, rose petals, and slippery elm to make a soothing honey pastille.

Sassafras root barks are more aromatic, drying, and spicy than its leaves. Use them to make chai with burdock, sarsaparilla, spicebush, and wild ginger. Use the root bark in an aromatic bitters blend with aspen bark and tulip poplar twigs.

Future Harvests

Sassafras is abundant and easily propagated by cuttings, seedlings, or suckers. You can gather handfuls of leaves from medium-sized trees without harming them. Gather the roots from saplings.

HERBAL PREPARATIONS

Sassafras leaf tea
Cold infusion
Drink 1 cup as needed.

Sassafras root tea
Hot infusion
Drink 1 cup as needed.

Sassafras root tincture
1 part fresh root bark, chopped
2 parts menstruum (95 percent alcohol, 5 percent distilled water)
Take 15–20 drops as needed.

---

self-heal

Prunella vulgaris

PARTS USED flowers, leaves

Self-heal may be small in stature, but it is a hugely valuable medicinal plant to use for healing wounds of all sorts, from sore throats, to ulcers, to burns.

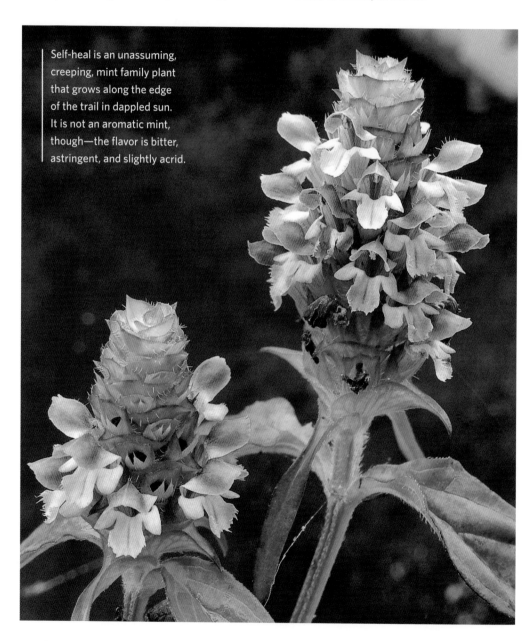

Self-heal is an unassuming, creeping, mint family plant that grows along the edge of the trail in dappled sun. It is not an aromatic mint, though—the flavor is bitter, astringent, and slightly acrid.

How to Identify

Self-heal is a creeping perennial mint that grows to 12 inches tall along the edges of trails in the dappled sun. Its small, deep green, lance-shaped leaves are serrated and distinctly veined, arranged oppositely on a square and reddish stem. Two-lipped flowers appear in the early summer; the top lip is hooded and purple, and the bottom lip is usually white, with fringed edges on the middle of three lobes. Self-heal's flavor is bitter, astringent, and slightly acrid.

Where, When, and How to Wildcraft

Wildcraft the leaves and flowers when the plant begins to bloom in early summer. Gather a few leaves and flowers by hand from each plant. Prepare them fresh or dry them for later use.

Medicinal Uses

Self-heal helps facilitate tissue- and wound-healing. Prepare it as a tea with echinacea, plantain, and slippery elm to treat a sore throat or to use as a mouth gargle to dry up mouth ulcers. A tea of self-heal and plantain can also be incorporated in a healing protocol to address ulcerative issues of the digestive tract, including stomach ulcers and diverticulitis.

Use self-heal tea as a topical wound wash to astringe burns and minor scrapes and abrasions. To stanch bleeding in minor cuts, combine self-heal and yarrow for a field poultice. The plant can also be infused in oil to create a healing skin salve.

Future Harvests

Gather a few leaves and flowers by hand from each plant, taking care not to remove too many, to avoid inhibiting the plant's ability to photosynthesize and reproduce.

HERBAL PREPARATIONS

Self-heal tea
Infusion
Drink ¼ cup, or use topically as a wound wash, gargle, or poultice.

Self-heal–infused oil
1 part fresh flowers and leaves, chopped
2 parts oil
Use for massage.

shepherd's purse

Capsella bursa-pastoris
PARTS USED leaves, seedpods, stems

*Shepherd's purse is a traditional plant medicine used to
astringe weepy wounds and stanch bleeding.*

How to Identify

A member of the mustard
family, shepherd purse has a
slender, hairy, branching stalk
that grows to about 18 inches
from a rosette of heavily lobed
and pointed leaves. Leaves are
2–6 inches long and variable
in shape along the stalk. Small
white flowers bloom throughout
the summer and develop into
flat, heart-shaped seedpods in
early summer. It's a rough and
dry plant to the touch with an
acrid and astringent taste.

Where, When, and How to Wildcraft

You'll find this unassuming and
self-sowing petite annual weed
growing in even the poorest
soils along sidewalks, in parking
lots, in weedy gardens, and in
urban lots. Gather the entire
plant at any time; it pulls easily
from the soil. Gather the seedpods in early summer. Prepare
the leaves, seedpods, and stems
fresh or dry them for later use.

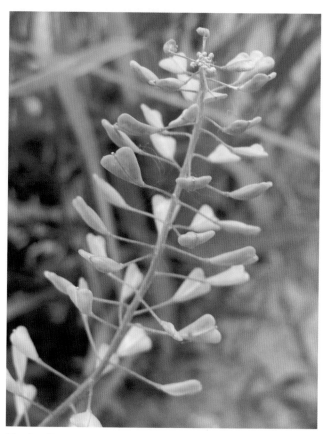

Shepherd's purse is traditionally known for its ability to stanch
bleeding in first aid situations and can help heal wounded,
prolapsed skin.

Medicinal Uses

Use shepherd's purse internally or externally.
Prepare a decoction to drink as tea to soothe
internal wounds from stomach ulcers and
diverticulitis. Consider adding plantain and
self-heal as well. Externally, use shepherd's
purse to help heal wounded skin, clean a
wound, and stanch bleeding. Add echinacea,
plantain, and self-heal to facilitate healing
and prevent septic infection. For mouth

ulcers, prepare shepherd's purse as a mouth gargle to astringe and tone oral tissues. Midwives have long integrated shepherd's purse into their birthing kits, offering it to new mothers to assist with postpartum bleeding.

Future Harvests

Shepherd's purse is a common, self-sowing weed and can be safely gathered without affecting future harvests.

Cautions, Concerns, and Considerations

Shepherd's purse grows abundantly in waste places and in disturbed soils. Gather your harvest in an area that is clean and free of potential contaminants (particularly in urban lots).

HERBAL PREPARATIONS

Shepherd's purse tea
Infusion
Drink ¼ cup, or use topically as a wound wash or mouth gargle.

Shepherd's purse tincture
1 part fresh leaves, seedpods, and stems, chopped
2 parts menstruum (50 percent alcohol, 50 percent distilled water)
Take 10–15 drops as needed.

skullcap

Scutellaria species
blisswort, blue skullcap, mad-dog skullcap
PARTS USED flowers, leaves, stems

Skullcap is an unassuming woodland plant for the home apothecary that can be used to make a relaxant tea or tincture.

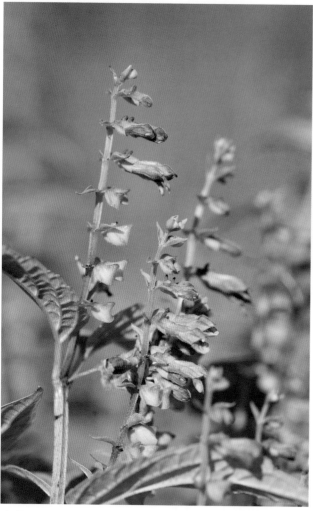

Skullcap derives its name from the caplike appearance of the outer whorl of its small purple flowers. While not a sedative like valerian or California poppy, skullcap can help relax tension and nourish the nervous system.

How to Identify

Skullcap is a vibrant green plant in the mint family. Growing 3–5 feet tall, its square stems are tinged in purple. Leaves grow in an opposite arrangement on the stem and are serrated, veined, ovate, and about 2–3 inches in length. Tubular purple flowers bloom in midsummer, with a petite protuberance atop each blossom. The entire plant lacks aroma and is slightly soapy in flavor.

Where, When, and How to Wildcraft

Look for skullcap growing in shady woods, thickets, and along roadsides in wet ditches. Gather the flowers, leaves, and stems from spring until mid- to late summer when the plant finishes blooming.

Use skullcap flowers, leaves, and stems fresh, or dry them for later use. Because the plant parts dry down significantly to a very small amount of dry herbs, fresh plant preparations of tincture are a more sustainable way to use skullcap.

Medicinal Uses

Though it is not as sedating as valerian, skullcap can help relax tension and nourish the nervous system. It works especially well for people who are overly rigid in temperament.

Use skullcap as a tea or tincture alone or with other herbs such as ashwagandha (*Withania somnifera*), blue vervain, lemon balm, passionflower, and rose. Skullcap is also useful in the first aid kit as a pain-reliever. For trauma and injury with excessive pain, blend skullcap with valerian. For muscle cramping or dull-achy pain, blend skullcap with black cohosh and crampbark in a tea or tincture.

Future Harvests

Skullcap does not grow prolifically through-out the Midwest. Hand-gather only a few leaves and flowers from each plant to maintain future harvests.

HERBAL PREPARATIONS

Skullcap tea
Decoction
Drink ¼ cup as needed.

Skullcap tincture
1 part fresh flowers and leaves, chopped
2 parts menstruum (50 percent alcohol, 50 percent distilled water)
Take 25 drops as needed.

slippery elm

Ulmus rubra
red elm
PARTS USED inner bark

Slippery elm's mucilaginous inner bark can be prepared as a medicine to bring moisture to and soothe inflamed and dried tissues of the respiratory system, digestive tract, and skin.

How to Identify
Slippery elm is a grand tree, growing to 60 feet or more at maturity. Its gray bark is deeply furrowed, and its branches extend across the top of the tree canopy. Leaves are oblong, 4–8 inches long, rough above and velvety underneath, with doubly serrated margins and deep veins. The most notable identifier of slippery elm is its mucilaginous, or slimy, white inner bark, which can be dried and used medicinally. After flowering in the early spring, the tree produces ½ to ¾ inch winged samaras that each contain a single seed.

Where, When, and How to Wildcraft
Look for slippery elm in mixed hardwood forests and along river or stream banks. Large and valuable older trees are also cultivated in yards and parks and around public buildings.

In the early spring, harvest branches of slippery elm to access the soft, white inner bark. Strip off the exterior hardwood, and then strip off long pieces of the inner bark with a sharp knife. Lay the inner bark pieces on a tarp to dry in the shade. When they are dry, cut the strips into pieces and store them in an airtight container.

Medicinal Uses
Slippery elm is one of the most useful plants for an herbalist. With its mucilaginous

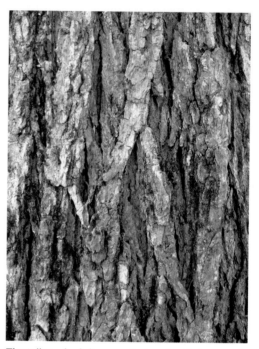

The tall trunk of slippery elm has deeply furrowed, gray bark.

properties, the inner bark is used to soothe and moisturize inflamed and dried tissues.

An infusion of slippery elm can help soothe sore throats, ease a dry and congested respiratory system, and heal dry and ulcerated tissues of the digestive tract. Herbs that work well in combination with slippery elm include plantain and rose, as well as mullein and wild cherry bark for dry respiratory conditions.

Dry slippery elm bark can be ground and prepared as a useful and soothing throat drop made with honey, or it can be combined with equal parts powdered licorice root, rose petal, and sage. These drops can soothe a dry, scratchy throat and can facilitate expectoration of stuck mucus in the lungs.

Future Harvests

Slippery elm trees can be killed by the Dutch elm disease fungus, *Ceratocystis ulmi*, which is spread by elm bark beetles. These tiny, dark-brown beetles live between the bark and the wood on diseased and dying elm trees. To avoid spreading the disease, prune the branches from healthy trees that show no symptoms. (Symptoms include one or more wilted branches, or branches with yellow leaves when the rest of the tree looks healthy.)

To help ensure that the fungus is not transmitted from tree-to-tree, do not transport cut wood or slabs of bark, which might contain beetles and the fungus. Strip the inner bark from cut branches onsite and keep the bark contained until you get back home for processing.

Cautions, Concerns, and Considerations

Cutting and burning diseased trees is the most common way communities try to control Dutch elm disease, though fungicide injection is sometimes used for urban trees that are particularly valuable. Because the fungicides used may be harmful to humans,

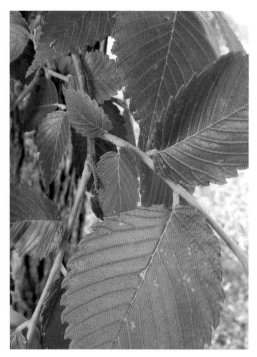

Slippery elm leaves are doubly serrated and asymmetrical.

avoid collecting wind-fallen or arborist-pruned branches in those areas. At the very least, contact your local forestry department to find out if particular trees have been treated.

HERBAL PREPARATIONS

Slippery elm tea
Cool water infusion
Drink 1 cup as needed.

Solomon's seal

Polygonatum biflorum
PARTS USED rhizomes

Solomon's seal is an excellent field medicine and herbal apothecary staple for musculoskeletal injuries and joint pain that comes from trauma, overuse, or acute degeneration of the joints, tendons, and ligaments.

How to Identify

The zig-zagging stalks of Solomon's seal grow 1–3 feet tall and droop gracefully with the weight of leaves and berries in the summertime. The leaves of this perennial (to 4 inches long) are bright green, smooth, parallel-veined, and arranged alternately along the stem.

Small and showy green-yellow or white flowers dangle from each leaf axil and are replaced in the fall by ½ inch berries that range in color from green to black. The plant is easy to identify in winter, because its sturdy stalks often hold onto its berries. It is a favorite for deer to munch on, especially in urban areas where there is little open space for them to roam and gather food.

The thin, white, and knobby rhizome is about ½ to ¾ inch in diameter.

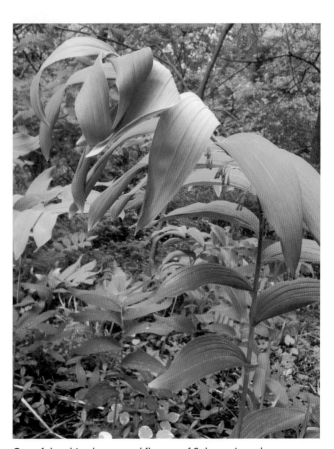

Graceful arching leaves and flowers of Solomon's seal.

Frequently, false Solomon's seal (*Maianthemum racemosum*) is mistaken for true Solomon's seal (*Polygonatum biflorum*), because of false Solomon's seal's similar erect, branching stalks and leaves that alternate on the stem. A differentiating factor is the arrangement of flowers and berries. False Solomon's seal has a white terminal flower plume at the top of the stem that produces bright red berries in midsummer, as opposed to the dangling flowers and berries of true Solomon's seal. The roots of false Solomon's seal are also edible, however, and can be used similarly to the rhizomes of the true Solomon's seal.

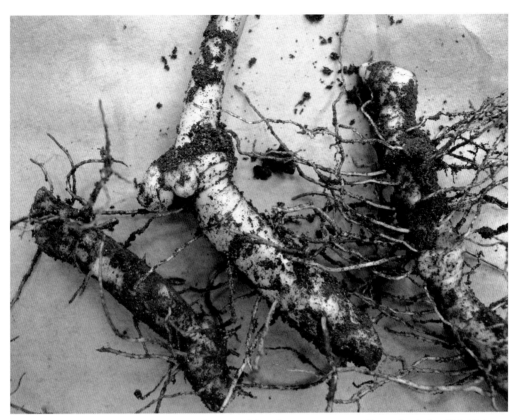

Solomon's seal rhizomes can be prepared as a poultice, tincture, massage oil, or salve to heal joint injuries. As a liniment or a fresh plant compress it can help reduce tissue damage assuming that no ligament is completely torn.

Where, When, and How to Wildcraft

Solomon's seal grows in woodland shade in moist or wet soils. In some areas, you'll find it growing abundantly in large stands, where it carpets the ground.

Gather new shoots when they emerge in early spring. Once the shoots are up, or if you can find a stalk from last year, you'll find it easy to locate and sustainably harvest the rhizome, which you can gather at any time.

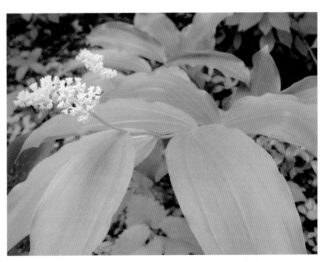

Flowers of false Solomon's seal are held in terminal clusters above the stem, unlike the dangling blossoms of true Solomon's seal.

Joint Injuries: There Are Herbs for That

Most joint injuries come with compensatory muscle tension and tightness. You can combine Solomon's seal with herbs such as catnip, crampbark, and valerian to relax muscles. With bursitis, add goldenrod to help alleviate excess fluid and swelling. With other skeletal alignment issues, add mullein roots and leaves. For trauma with sharp, shooting nerve pain, pair Solomon's seal with St. John's wort.

Damaged and dry musculoskeletal tissues and joints require healthy fats, collagen, vitamin A, and other nutrients to be healthy and pliable. Internal use of Solomon's seal as a tincture can help facilitate the assimilation and delivery of these nutrients from the gut to the tissues. Supporting healthy digestion is a key in healing damaged and dry musculoskeletal tissues before they become chronic arthritis.

To gather the rhizomes sustainably, locate two adjacent stems of the plant and seek out (with a small fork or digging tool) the connecting rhizome segment. Slice off the middle segment between the plants, leaving sufficient rhizomes on the main stalks so that both will stay rooted in the soil. Prepare the rhizomes fresh or dry them for later use.

Medicinal Uses

Solomon's seal helps to nourish and deliver moisture to the tissues of the joints and can help correct for overly dry fascia, tendons, and ligaments that are tight and constricted.

Prepare Solomon's seal as a poultice, tincture, massage oil, or salve. For trauma to a joint, use it as a liniment or a fresh plant compress to reduce tissue damage (assuming the ligament is not torn). A Solomon's seal–infused massage oil or salve can work similarly and is useful to incorporate into a recovery routine for athletes who commonly face overuse injuries from training.

Future Harvests

Gathering Solomon's seal rhizomes on a regular basis could put a strain on the plant population (even if only the middle rhizomes are gathered). The plant can be propagated by root cuttings and is a nice addition to a woodland or permaculture landscape plan.

HERBAL PREPARATIONS

Solomon's seal tincture
1 part fresh rhizomes, chopped
2 parts menstruum (50 percent alcohol,
  50 percent distilled water)
Take 15–25 drops as needed.

Solomon's seal–infused oil
1 part fresh rhizomes, chopped
2 parts oil
Use for massage.

spearmint

Mentha spicata

PARTS USED flowers, leaves

*Gather spearmint for the apothecary to create soothing and aromatic teas
or tinctures. Because of its relaxant nature, spearmint tea can soothe upset
stomachs and sore throats.*

How to Identify

Spearmint is a creeping perennial that grows
4–5 feet tall. Green, lance-shaped, toothed
leaves are oppositely arranged on square
stems. Small and white, pale violet, or pink
flower heads are produced on slender spikes
in late summer, after which the plant dries
significantly and begins to die back.

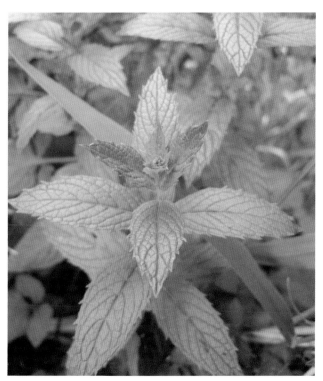

The flavor of spearmint is slightly different from that of its cousin
peppermint. Spearmint is a less spicy and more cooling, relaxing
herb; as a tea it is even gentle enough for wee ones.

Where, When, and How to Wildcraft

Look for spearmint in woodlands, growing
alongside stream banks and creeks. Like peppermint, spearmint grows wild in moist, well-
drained soil in partial sun. It is tender and
more aromatic in midspring and becomes
rougher and spicier as the weather warms.
Spearmint flavor is slightly different from
that of peppermint—it's less
spicy and more cooling.

Wildcraft the plant when
it is 1–3 feet tall and before it
flowers for the choicest leaves
and flavors. Leaves can be gathered and used throughout the
season, however; use your nose
and taste buds to determine
flavor and quality.

Store the fresh flowers and
leaves in the refrigerator for up
to a week, wrapped in a moist
towel. To ensure maximum
aromatics, after gathering full
stems of spearmint, bundle
them and dry the entire plant.
Store dried flowers and leaves in
an airtight container to preserve them for later use.

Medicinal Uses

Spearmint is particularly
useful as a relaxant herb.
Spearmint tea gently soothes

upset stomachs and sore throats; it is gentle enough to use for children. Drinking a cup of spearmint tea before bedtime can help ease away the day's stresses.

Future Harvests

Spearmint spreads readily via underground rhizomes, and gathering its stalks will not affect the plant's future growth and harvest.

HERBAL PREPARATIONS

Spearmint tea
Infusion
Drink ½ cup as needed.

Spearmint leaf tincture
1 part fresh leaves, chopped
2 parts menstruum (50 percent alcohol,
    50 percent distilled water)
or
1 part dry leaves, chopped
4 parts menstruum (50 percent alcohol,
    50 percent distilled water)
Take 15 drops as needed.

spicebush

Lindera benzoin
PARTS USED berries, leaves, twigs

The aromatic berries of spicebush can be used in warming teas and tinctures. This herb is included in blends to soothe digestive issues and in topical massage blends for muscle rubs.

How to Identify
Spicebush is a small deciduous tree, 6–15 feet in height and spread. The brown to gray-brown bark is speckled with light-colored lenticels. Leaves are smooth, oblong, and veined, arranged alternately on the branches. When crushed, the leaves emit a strong, spicy odor similar to that of allspice. Yellow-green flower clusters form in early spring, followed by bright red, ⅜ inch fruits (drupes) in late summer. The bark, leaves, and fruit are all aromatic.

Where, When, and How to Wildcraft
Look for spicebush growing in moist locations in woods, ravines, valleys, and along streams and hedgerows in partial sun. Wildcraft the leaves and twigs at any time. Harvest the berries in the late summer and fall.

Before storing, make sure that the plant material is entirely dry. Use a dehydrator to dry the berries before storing them in an airtight container that will preserve their aromatics. Dried twigs can be powdered in

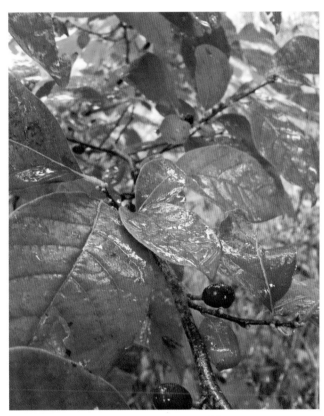

Spicebush is a native herb with a scent and flavor reminiscent of tropical allspice. Its berries, leaves, and twigs are aromatic and warming.

a spice grinder; use a mortar and pestle to crush dried berries and leaves.

Medicinal Uses
Spicebush berries, leaves, and twigs are spicy, aromatic, and warming. They are useful in

the home apothecary to support healthy circulation. They help drive the blood to the extremities, which is useful on cold winter days or at the onset of a cold or flu with fever.

Use spicebush to flavor a warming foraged chai blend with burdock, sarsaparilla, and sassafras. Add it to decoctions of reishi and other medicinal mushrooms to lend warming and aromatic flavors to tea. Use spicebush in blends of elderberry syrup where cinnamon or allspice might be used.

Tincture of spicebush can be prepared to use in bitters blends to support digestion as a gas-relieving carminative. Combine spicebush with aspen bark to add a dynamic dry, warming note. It also works well with lemon balm, tulip poplar bark, and other metabolic tonics such as burdock, ceanothus, and yellow dock.

Infuse spicebush in oil to use for a warming massage. Combine it with cayenne, goldenrod, turmeric, and wild ginger in an oil rub that stimulates circulation and eases muscle aches and pains.

Future Harvests

You can gather spicebush berries, leaves, and twigs without significantly impacting future harvests. It is propagated by cuttings and is a good plant to add to a permaculture landscape in areas that receive partial or no sun.

HERBAL PREPARATIONS

Spicebush tea
Infusion
Drink ¼ cup as needed.

Spicebush tincture
1 part fresh berries
2 parts menstruum (50 percent alcohol, 50 percent distilled water)
Take 10–15 drops as needed.

Spicebush-infused oil
1 part fresh berries
2 parts oil
Use for massage.

spotted bee balm

Monarda punctata

dotted mint, spotted horsemint

PARTS USED flowers, leaves, stems

Make no mistake: the delicate blossoms of spotted bee balm are not delicate at all! These spicy and aromatic beauties are useful in teas for colds and flus and are a powerful antimicrobial for wounds and burns.

How to Identify

Spotted bee balm is a perennial native plant in the mint family. Typically 6–8 inches tall, it can grow up to 3 feet tall in the best conditions—well-drained or sandy soils in full sun. Clumps of plants are connected by runners. Leaves are arranged oppositely on square stems and are slightly toothed and hairy. Its two-lipped flowers grow in tiers that surround the stem and are quite showy—creamy white and yellow with lilac spots—with several large pink, leafy bracts clustered below each tier of blossoms.

Where, When, and How to Wildcraft

Collect leaves and wildcraft stems of spotted bee balm at any time; both can be prepared and used fresh or dried for later use. In mid- to late summer, gather a few stalks, leaving some for the butterflies and honey bees to enjoy. Bundle the stalks and dry them for use as tea. Store all fully dry plant material in airtight containers to preserve the aromatics.

Medicinal Uses

Spotted bee balm's healing properties truly shine when it is brewed as hot tea. Its warming aromatics dispel the damp chill of a rainy day, stimulate circulation in cold hands and feet, and soothe those suffering with fever and chills. Use a tincture of spotted bee balm similarly by taking large dropperfuls at the onset of cold or flu. Or add it to a basic elderberry elixir.

To clear sinuses, use the flowers and leaves as a steam inhalation. The aroma from the steaming pot can also help clear rooms of stagnant wintertime air.

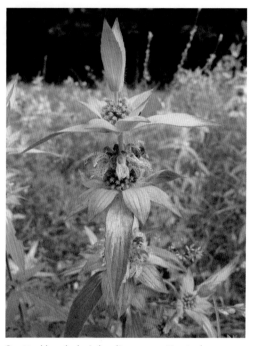

Spotted bee balm's healing properties truly shine when it is brewed as a hot tea. Its warming aromatics dispel the damp chill of a rainy day, stimulate circulation in cold hands and feet, and soothe anyone suffering fever and chills.

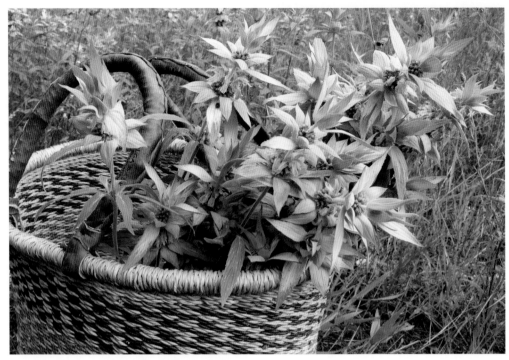

The fresh spring leaves and stems of spotted bee balm can be wildcrafted anytime and prepared fresh or dried. The flowering stalks can be wildcrafted in midsummer, bundled, and dried for use as tea in the winter.

Like the related wild bergamot (*Monarda fistulosa*), spotted bee balm has excellent antimicrobial properties. Infuse its fresh flowers and leaves in honey to create a topical ointment for burns and fungal infections. It can also be prepared as a topical wash to clean and dry wounds.

Future Harvests

Cut only a portion of the plant to use for tea and allow some blossoms to go to seed. This is an easy-to-grow perennial that can be propagated by runners, cuttings, and transplants in the fall.

HERBAL PREPARATIONS

Spotted bee balm tea
Infusion
Drink ½ cup, or use for a wound wash or steam inhalation.

Spotted bee balm tincture
1 part fresh flowers and leaves, chopped
2 parts menstruum (50 percent alcohol, 50 percent distilled water)
or
1 part dry flowers and leaves, chopped
4 parts menstruum (50 percent alcohol, 50 percent distilled water)
Take 15–25 drops as needed.

Spotted bee balm–infused honey
1 part fresh flowers and leaves, chopped
3 parts raw, unpasteurized honey
Use as needed.

spruce

Picea species
PARTS USED bark, branch tips, needles, resin, shoots

Spruce needles and resins are useful in medicinal teas and salves.
Not only are the needles rich in vitamin C, but when used in an aromatic
steam inhalation, they can clear stuffy sinus congestion from winter colds.

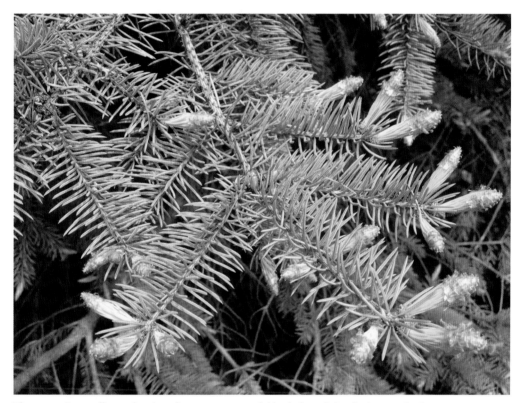

The aromatic needles and resins of spruce are a useful herbal medicine for teas and salves.

How to Identify

Spruce is a coniferous evergreen 60–200 feet tall. The bark is thin, dark gray-brown, and somewhat scaly. Branches grow in a whorled pattern, with single bluish needles attached in a spiral fashion at right angles to the branch. When needles are shed, they leave behind little pegs that make the twigs and branches feel rough.

Where, When, and How to Wildcraft

Look for spruce trees growing in moist soils along stream banks and other water sources. The conifer is common in wild as well as urban landscapes, and it is often used as a holiday tree. The new tips and shoots in the early spring are choice to gather for medicine-making.

Collect needles by hand at any time; they are most tender and aromatic in the spring, which is also the best time to collect bark and resin. To gather the bark, trim the small twigs and branches to use in teas or tinctures. Scrape the resin from the sides of the tree, and store it in a sealed container to use for salve.

Medicinal Uses

To make an excellent steam inhalation to clear sinus congestion, add boiling water to a pot with fresh or dry needles, cover, and let steep for 3 to 5 minutes. To make an aromatic tea, sweeten the infusion with honey.

Spruce is markedly resinous. The young bark and resin can be extracted in high-proof alcohol to make a healing tincture used similarly to bee propolis to care for wounds and sore throats. Spruce resin is a useful first aid remedy to use in the field to cover scrapes and cuts. Or use it to cover canker sores in the mouth.

Spruce resin infused in olive oil can be used alone as an aromatic massage oil or prepared as a salve with beeswax. The salve is helpful to prevent skin chafing and windburn.

Future Harvests

Harvest branches, needles, and bark in a sustainable manner. Because spruce is a common tree, gathering these plant parts in moderation will not impact future harvests.

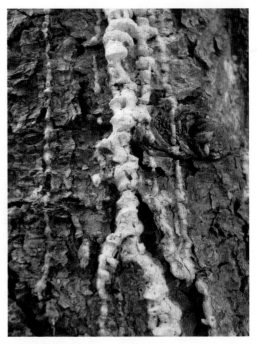

Spruce resin contains aromatic oils that are helpful in healing wounds.

HERBAL PREPARATIONS

Spruce needle and branch tip tea
Infusion
Drink ½ cup as needed, use for a wound wash, or prepare as a steam inhalation.

Spruce needle tincture
1 part fresh needles, chopped
2 parts menstruum (95 percent alcohol, 5 percent distilled water)
Take 10–15 drops as needed.

Spruce needle-infused oil
1 part fresh needles, chopped
2 parts oil
Use for massage.

St. John's wort

Hypericum perforatum
PARTS USED flowers, leaves

St. John's wort, known by many as a common health food store supplement, has a wide range of uses as a field medicine and apothecary herb for pain and wound care.

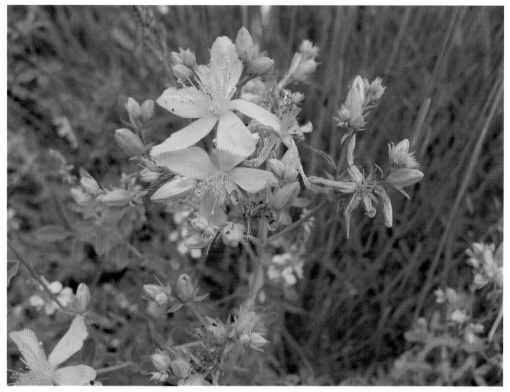

St. John's wort blooms from the summer solstice through late summer. Because of its sunny disposition and its aromatic smell, St. John's wort is useful in clearing melancholy and sadness.

How to Identify

St. John's wort is an herbaceous perennial that grows 24–36 inches tall. It has oppositely arranged, stalkless, narrow, and oblong green leaves, ½ to 1 inch in length, that are covered with translucent dots of glandular tissue. When held up to the light, the leaves appear to be perforated, which gave rise to the plant's species name.

St. John's wort blooms near the summer solstice in late June. Small, yellow, five-petal blossoms are covered with small, black glandular dots on the petal tips and sepals. The flower releases a reddish colored oil when crushed between the fingers and is slightly fragrant.

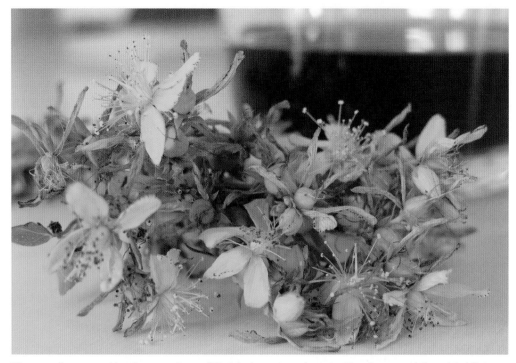

The open flowers and tender green tops of St. John's wort can be cut with scissors and then dried flat on screens for tea or prepared fresh for herbal remedies.

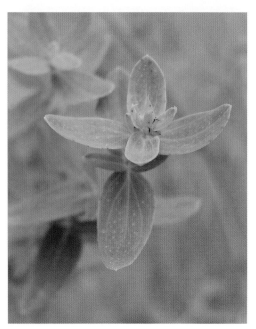

St. John's wort leaves shine with translucent pin-pricks when held up to the light.

Where, When, and How to Wildcraft

Look for St. John's wort growing in sunny open fields and disturbed waste places. Harvest the open flowers and tender green leaves in summer, and then dry them flat on screens for tea or prepare them to use fresh. The plant can bloom successively throughout the summer and offers the forager multiple harvests across the season.

Medicinal Uses

St. John's wort can be prepared in a number of medicinal remedies, including an infused oil or a plant extract in vodka. Both preparations are dark red in color, the result of the hypericin in the plant, which is one of its main medicinal constituents.

Used as a pain remedy, St. John's wort is helpful for injuries with sharp, shooting pain, such as bone breaks, strains, sprains, sciatica, carpal tunnel, and nerve pain. Apply it as a poultice to treat acute pain (good to know as an emergency field medicine) or topically as a tincture or infused oil. The topical oil also offers relief for chronic pain caused by fibromyalgia or rheumatoid arthritis. St. John's wort works well with goldenrod, mullein, and yarrow to help with chronic pain and musculoskeletal injuries.

St. John's wort is also effective in lifting melancholy. Sipping an aromatic tea infusion can elevate your mood, and the tea is perfect for the middle of winter, when many folks suffer from seasonal affective disorder. It pairs well with chamomile, hawthorn, and lemon balm for relief from melancholy and sadness.

Future Harvests

St. John's wort is considered a noxious weed in some areas of the Midwest. Gathering the flowers and leaves of this perennial plant will not significantly impact future harvests.

 ## Cautions, Concerns, and Considerations

Those who use pharmaceutical blood thinners such as warfarin (Coumadin) are advised to avoid use of St. John's wort, which can interfere with the body's ability to process the drug. Using St. John's wort can also cause photodermatitis (a rash resulting from sun exposure) in some people. If this occurs, discontinue use internally and topically.

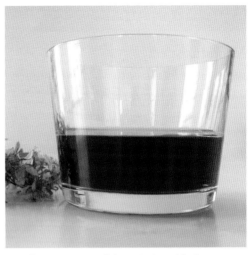

St. John's wort is useful in injuries with sharp, shooting pain. Its deep red oil is also known to offer relief for chronic pain caused by fibromyalgia and rheumatoid arthritis.

HERBAL PREPARATIONS

St. John's wort tea
Infusion
Drink ½ cup as needed, or use topically as a wound wash.

St. John's wort tincture
1 part fresh flowers and leaves, chopped
2 parts menstruum (50 percent alcohol, 50 percent distilled water)
or
1 part dry flowers and leaves, chopped
4 parts menstruum (50 percent alcohol, 50 percent distilled water)
Take 25–30 drops as needed.

St. John's wort–infused oil
1 part fresh flowers and leaves
2 parts oil
Use for massage.

sweet clover

Melilotus species

white sweet clover (*M. alba*), yellow sweet clover (*M. officinalis*)

PARTS USED flowers, leaves

Sweet clover's heady notes of vanilla and honey waft through the air and can be captured for use as a mood-uplifting, space-clearing herb, very handy during the depths of the dark winter months.

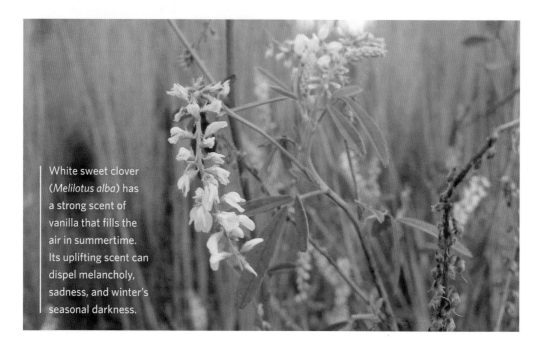

White sweet clover (*Melilotus alba*) has a strong scent of vanilla that fills the air in summertime. Its uplifting scent can dispel melancholy, sadness, and winter's seasonal darkness.

How to Identify

Sweet clover is an herbaceous biennial plant that grows 4–6 feet tall. Its dull green, smooth stem is erect and branched. Trifoliate, oval leaves alternate along the stem. Small, sweet-scented flower clusters are white (*M. alba*) or yellow (*M. officinalis*) and bloom in spring and summer, going to seed shortly thereafter. Seedpods and are broad, black, and wrinkled, and each pod contains one seed. The entire plant smells distinctly of mowed grass and vanilla and tastes somewhat bitter.

Where, When, and How to Wildcraft

Look for sweet clover growing in ditches, dry fields, prairies, along roadsides, and in waste places. Sweet clover is used as a common cover crop to fix nitrogen in the soil, but it also grows in other areas of poor soil quality. Because it grows abundantly and readily escapes from cultivation, it is considered a noxious weed in some areas.

Wildcraft sweet clover leaves and flowers in full bloom on a dry, sunny summer day. Process the blossoms and leaves immediately or dry them for later use. To dry an entire stalk, hang it in a cool, dry place with good ventilation so it does not mold.

Medicinal Uses

Sweet clover is a special plant for the herbal apothecary, because its uplifting scent can dispel melancholy, sadness, and seasonal doldrums. Adding bundles of dried sweet clover to your home's decor provides attractive dried flower arrangements that emit sweet summer aromas throughout the winter months.

To prepare a refreshing aromatic mist, make a tincture of fresh sweet clover flowers and leaves, dilute it with distilled water, and pour it into a spray bottle. Spritz the cooling mist on the skin and face.

Future Harvests

Sweet clover is a beneficial plant in the garden, with nitrogen-fixing root nodes that can improve poor soils, but because it is a voracious spreader, it has been labeled a noxious weed by many native plant folk. Gathering the plant by the armful will do little to impact future harvests or the plant's sustainability.

 Cautions, Concerns, and Considerations

Because of its chemical compounds, which include the presence of warfarin, those using pharmaceutical blood thinners such as Coumadin should avoid working with and consuming sweet clover.

HERBAL PREPARATIONS

Sweet clover tincture
1 part fresh flowers and leaves
2 parts menstruum (50 percent alcohol, 50 percent distilled water)
Use topically as a facial mist, or use as a room spray.

---

teasel

Dipsacus sylvestris

PARTS USED roots

Teasel is used to heal and nourish torn tissues such as tendons and ligaments and can also be used as a part of a healing protocol for Lyme disease.

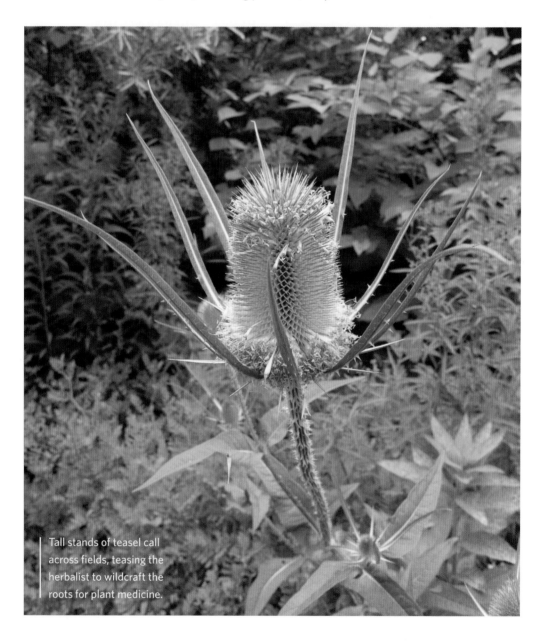

Tall stands of teasel call across fields, teasing the herbalist to wildcraft the roots for plant medicine.

How to Identify

Teasel is a nonnative biennial plant that grows 4–8 feet tall. In the plant's first year, ovate, hairy leaves form a basal rosette, 4–6 inches wide. Thick, prickly stems grow from the base of the plant in its second year, with toothed, lanceolate leaves, 8–16 inches long, which wrap around the stalk. A row of small spines line the underside of each leaf midrib.

In midsummer, an oblong terminal inflorescence of small pink or purple flowers forms atop a basal whorl of long, spiny bracts. The flower head dries to a coarse, bristly seed head in late fall that can hang on to the plant throughout the winter months.

Teasel roots are white, spindly, and not aromatic.

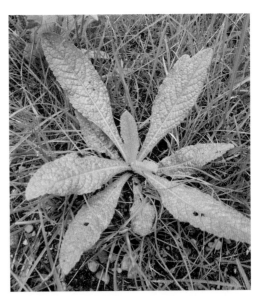

The first year basal rosette of teasel. Harvest the roots at the end of the first year, before it sends up its flower stalk in the second year.

Where, When, and How to Wildcraft

Teasel thrives in disturbed soil, and you'll find it growing in open fields, empty lots, and woodland edges. Gather the roots from basal rosettes of first-year plants in the late fall, before the plants send up flower stalks in the second year.

Using a garden fork, dig the spiny rosettes from the ground. Then, wearing gloves to avoid the prickles, sort through the rosettes, separating out any unwanted plants, and clip away the leaves from the roots and crowns of the plant. Scrub the roots to remove soil and debris, and then remove the crown and roughly chop the roots. Use teasel roots fresh in a tincture or salve or dry them for later use.

Medicinal Uses

Prepare teasel roots as a poultice, tincture, massage oil, or salve to help heal joint injuries. For joint trauma, prepare them as a liniment or a fresh compress to help reduce damage to the tissues (assuming no completely torn ligaments). A teasel salve or massage oil can work similarly and is useful to incorporate into a recovery routine for athletes who commonly face overuse injuries from training.

Because most joint injuries are accompanied by compensatory tension and tightness, you can combine teasel with catnip, crampbark, or valerian to relax the muscles. With bursitis, add goldenrod to help alleviate excess fluids and swelling. With other skeletal alignment issues, adding mullein root and leaf and Solomon's seal (especially when the tissues are stiff and unlubricated) is useful. For trauma with sharp, shooting nerve pain, add St. John's wort to improve the healing formula.

Damaged and dry musculoskeletal tissues and joints require healthy fats, collagen, and vitamin A, among other nutrients, to be healthy and pliable. Using a tincture of teasel and Solomon's seal can help facilitate the assimilation and delivery of these nutrients from the gut to the tissues.

Teasel roots are used as a part of a healing protocol for Lyme disease. Incorporate teasel

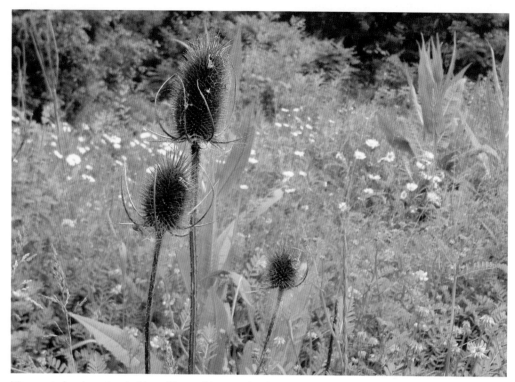

It's easy to locate a stand of teasel by seeking out the distinctive dry stalks topped with seed heads. Look at the ground next to the old stalks and you may see new teasel plants coming up.

root tincture into an overall treatment to help support the immune system. Because of the potentially debilitating effects of this disease, it is important to seek conventional medical treatment as soon as possible upon detecting an inflamed tick bite. You can use small-drop doses of teasel root tincture in tandem with conventional treatments (antibiotics are common in the first weeks of an acute infection) and then continue to use it beyond the initial course of antibiotics treatment.

Future Harvests

Teasel is considered a noxious weed throughout the Midwest. Gathering its roots will not significantly affect its distribution.

Cautions, Concerns, and Considerations

Teasel is commonly treated with herbicides to prevent its spread. Inquire about this before gathering in any area that may have been treated.

HERBAL PREPARATIONS

Teasel root tincture
1 part fresh roots, chopped
2 parts menstruum (95 percent alcohol, 5 percent distilled water)
Take 10 drops as needed.

Teasel root–infused oil
1 part fresh roots, chopped
2 parts oil
Use for massage.

Liriodendron tulipifera
tulip tree, yellow poplar
PARTS USED branch tips, flowers

Herbalists use tulip poplar to help stimulate stagnant digestion. The aromatic spicy notes in the plant extract are used as a layer in a bitters blend to offer a warming flavor and carminative effect that can soothe an upset stomach from overindulgence.

How to Identify

Tulip poplars are tall and large deciduous hardwoods. The tree's furrowed bark is dark gray or brown. Leaves are smooth, 3–5 inches wide, palmate, and lobed; they grow in an alternate arrangement. In spring, the tree's flowers are remarkable and resemble a tulip or a tea cup, with bright, showy, single blooms in green, yellow, and orange. The fruit is a 3-inch brown cone that develops in late fall and is a good marker for off-season identification. The flowers, new twigs, and branches have a delicate, clove-like flavor that works in bitters blends or as a nervine.

Where, When, and How to Wildcraft

Tulip poplars are distributed throughout the middle and southeastern parts of the Midwest. Look for them in sunny, mild, and temperate growing locations in moderately moist, well-drained soils. They are often used as landscape trees and for reforestation because of their rapid growth.

Gather new branch tips and flowers from late June to early July. A big summer thunderstorm or high winds can bring down a significant number of brittle branches with new branch tips and flowers. These are easiest to gather, particularly because many of the small branches and blooms on the tree are completely out of reach. Cut the new tips and flowers into small pieces to dry, or process them fresh into simple syrup and plant extracts.

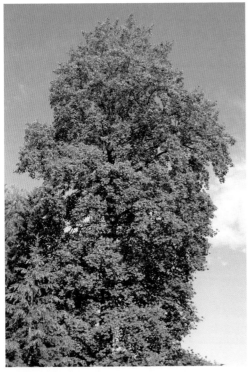

Mature tulip poplars can be more than 150 feet tall, with trunks up to 10 feet in diameter. The flowers, new twigs, and branches have a delicate, clove-like spice flavor that can be used in bitters blends or as a nervine.

Tree Medicine: Tulip Poplar Bitters Blend

Because of the tulip poplar's aromatic and spicy nature, herbalists use it to help stimulate stagnant digestion. The aromatic, spicy notes in the plant extract are great in a bitters blend, where they offer a warming flavor and carminative effect that can soothe an upset stomach resulting from overindulgence.

Use a high-proof alcohol to extract the resins of the plant. A locally made, spicy rum works delightfully well—the spiciness of the rum complements the spices of the plant.

To make a tulip poplar bitters blend, combine equal parts extracts of tulip poplar with basil, burdock, coffee, orange peel, and yellow dock. Sweeten the mixture with a bit of maple syrup or honey and bottle it in dropper bottles. Use 20–25 drops of this blend as needed to help soothe digestion, or use it liberally in cocktails or homemade sodas.

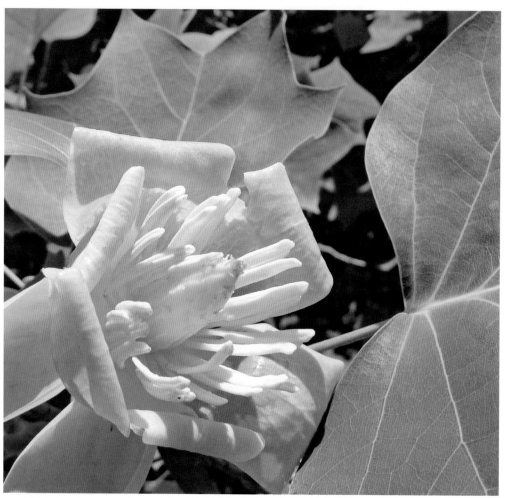

The flowers and tips of the branches have a warming spice flavor and make a useful culinary herb.

Medicinal Uses

The flowers and branch tips of tulip poplar have a warming, spicy flavor and make a useful culinary herb. Both are slightly resinous and can be dried or extracted into high-proof alcohol.

Teas or tinctures of tulip poplar can have a relaxing effect on the nervous system and are used as a skeletal muscle relaxant for those who are overstressed, to soothe a high-strung nervous system. Tulip poplar is most effective as a tincture in tea or water, because an infusion would not be as palatable and would bring out its more bitter notes.

Use tulip poplar tincture and salve to relax tight and tense muscles, particularly in the neck, back, and pelvic areas. A warm oil infusion of tulip poplar branch tips and flowers massaged on the lower back and lower abdominal area soothes menstrual cramps. It also works well as a post-workout massage oil to loosen tight muscles.

Future Harvests

The tulip poplar is a fast-growing hardwood, and gathering its fallen branches and flowers will do little to impact the tree's future harvests. The tree is easily propagated by cuttings.

HERBAL PREPARATIONS

Tulip poplar tincture

1 part fresh branch tips and flowers, chopped

2 parts menstruum (95 percent alcohol, 5 percent distilled water)

Take 15 drops as needed, or use topically as a muscle liniment.

Tulip poplar–infused oil

1 part fresh branch tips and flowers, chopped

2 parts oil

Use for massage.

turkey tail

Trametes versicolor
PARTS USED fruiting body

Turkey tail is deeply nutritive and nourishing to the immune system. A turkey tail broth is helpful for people who are convalescing after illness, because it is easy to digest and its nutrients are easily absorbed into the body.

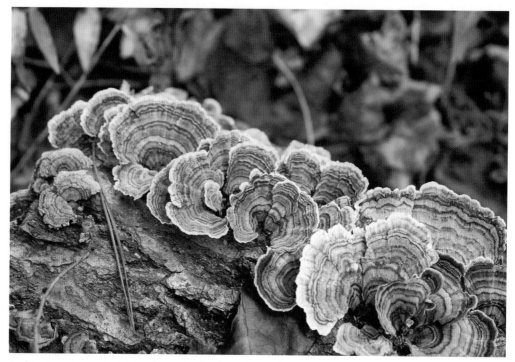

A ubiquitous fungus in Midwestern woodlands, turkey tail is deeply nutritive and nourishing to the immune system. Sip turkey tail tea at the onset of a cold, flu, or fever.

How to Identify

Turkey tail is a bracket fungus that grows in woodlands on decaying hardwood logs and stumps. The fruiting body is thin and flexible, and fuzzy or velvety on top, with vibrant, concentric rings of color ranging from brown, to red, orange, blue, and bright green. The color vibrancy is determined by the age of the fungus: the less vibrant the colors, the older the specimen.

On the white underside, large, visible pores contain spores. The porous underside of the fungus is one of the best ways to identify it in the field.

Where, When, and How to Wildcraft

Seek out fresh turkey tails in the spring and fall after a rain. Choose fresh fruiting bodies that are thin and flexible, rather than those that are brittle or rubbery. Cut them away from the host wood with a sharp knife, being careful not to remove the entire fungus from the wood. Coarsely chop the fungus into pieces, and dry the pieces on a screen or in a dehydrator.

Medicinal Uses

In Asia, specifically in traditional Chinese medicine, much research has demonstrated that turkey tail may have anticancer properties: the compounds in the fungus stimulate the immune system and affect tumor growth.

Turkey tail is high in polysaccharides and other compounds that are soluble only in water and cannot be extracted well in alcohol. Because of this, the easiest way to prepare and consume turkey tail is to combine the dry fungus in broths with herbs such as astragalus and burdock. Turkey tails have a neutral flavor and will not affect the flavor of the broth. Sip the medicinal broth at the onset of a cold, flu, or fever.

Future Harvests

Turkey tail grows in abundance throughout the Midwest. Gathering it for personal use will do little to impact future harvests of the plant. Take care, however, that you do not damage the fungal attachment when removing the fruiting body from the host wood, to ensure future harvests.

HERBAL PREPARATIONS

Turkey tail tea
Decoction
Drink ½ cup per day.

Arctostaphylos uva-ursi
bearberry, kinnikinnick
PARTS USED leaves

Uva-ursi is an evergreen creeping plant that is known an as aromatic and astringent medicine, useful in healing urinary tract infections.

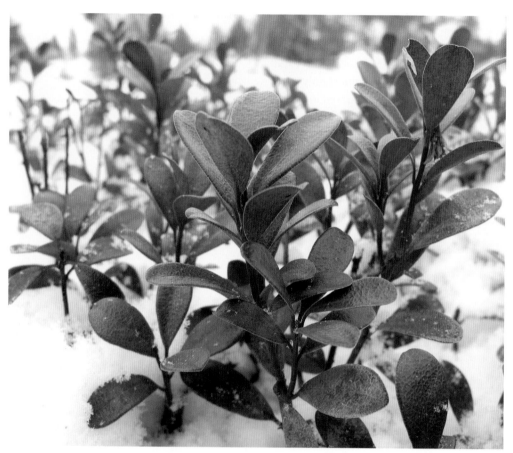

Uva-ursi is an aromatic and astringent plant. As a tea, it can be useful in treatments of chronic urinary tract infections, helping tone and astringe prolapsed and infected tissues.

How to Identify

Uva-ursi is a creeping evergreen plant that grows to about 24 inches tall. Arranged alternately along branching stems, the 1-inch-long, shiny, oblong leaves are smooth, leathery, and dark green, with a lighter, silver-gray color underneath. The leaves turn a dark red-purple in winter.

Throughout the summer, flowers develop in terminal clusters of petite, bell-shaped, pinkish or white blossoms. In late fall, red berries form and remain on the stem throughout the winter months.

Where, When, and How to Wildcraft

Look for uva-ursi growing in sandy soils in full sun in the Great Lakes dune areas, where it spreads prolifically, or in the sandy areas of the Midwest formed by glacial retreat. To wildcraft uva-ursi, gather the leaves at any time and use them fresh, or dry them for later use.

Medicinal Uses

Uva-ursi is an aromatic and astringent medicinal plant. As a tea, it is useful in treatments of chronic urinary tract infections, helping tone and astringe prolapsed and infected tissues. It pairs well with goldenrod, a plant that is equally astringent, and with cranberry in protocols to support the urinary tract.

Future Harvests

Uva-ursi is a common plant in some areas, but habitat loss has affected the plant. Carefully harvest the leaves, taking care not to strip the plant entirely, to ensure a healthy plant and future growth.

HERBAL PREPARATIONS

Uva-ursi tea
Infusion
Drink ½ cup per day.

Uva-ursi tincture
1 part fresh or dry leaves
2 parts menstruum (50 percent alcohol, 50 percent distilled water)
Take 15–20 drops as needed.

valerian

Valeriana officinalis
PARTS USED flowers, leaves

Valerian may have a strong odor similar to stinky socks, but it is a valuable and versatile plant medicine that can quell anxiety, reduce pain, stop muscle spasms, and induce sleep.

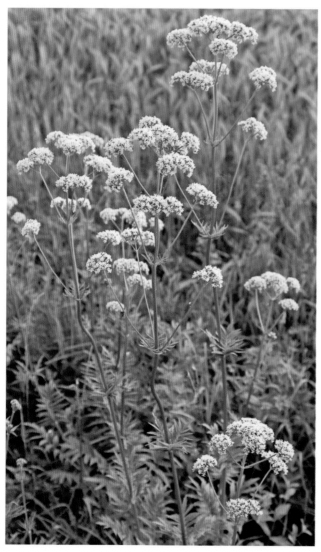

Valerian is a very useful nervine for the herbal apothecary. It is notably relaxant—even a sedative in certain persons.

How to Identify

Valerian is a perennial plant that grows to 4 feet tall in damp meadows, in full to dappled sun. Leaves are oppositely arranged, compound, and toothed, with some being whorled. The roots, leaves, and stems are notably aromatic with a skunky, resinous odor. Valerian blooms in midsummer, with clusters of sweet-smelling five-petaled tubular flowers that range in color from white to red.

Where, When, and How to Wildcraft

Look for valerian in damp meadows, and wildcraft it when the plant is in bloom in midsummer. Gather the stems with the flowers and leaves, which can be bundled and dried for later use or prepared fresh as a tincture, oil, or tea.

Medicinal Uses

Valerian is a useful nervine for the herbal apothecary. It is notably relaxant and can serve as a sedative for some people. For anxiety and insomnia, valerian blends well with lemon balm, passionflower, and skullcap for those who are highly anxious and need calming. These blends are also useful for calming emotional trauma in first aid situations.

Valerian is excellent in helping quell muscle spasms and ease tension in the body. Fresh or dry plant material can be extracted as an infused oil to use in massage or a salve for muscle tension, and a liniment of valerian plant extract can be used in this way as well.

Future Harvests

Gather the stems in moderation to ensure that the plant can produce seeds and continue to photosynthesize. Valerian is an easy plant to incorporate into a permaculture garden to help ensure future sustainable harvests.

Cautions, Concerns, and Considerations

Valerian can have an aggravating effect on some people. Try a small test dose of tincture or tea to make sure it is agreeable. After taking a few drops of tincture or tea, take time to notice whether you feel more agitation than relaxation. If you feel relaxed, the herb is suitable. If it causes aggravation, seek out an alternative sedative herb.

HERBAL PREPARATIONS

Valerian tea
Infusion
Drink ¼ cup as needed.

Valerian tincture
1 part fresh flowers and leaves, chopped
2 parts menstruum (95 percent alcohol, 5 percent distilled water)
or
1 part dry flowers and leaves, chopped
5 parts menstruum (95 percent alcohol, 5 percent distilled water)
Take 10–15 drops as needed.

Valerian-infused oil
1 part fresh flowers and leaves, chopped
2 parts olive or coconut oil
or
1 part dry flowers and leaves, chopped
4 parts olive or coconut oil
Use for massage.

Viola species

PARTS USED flowers, leaves

Violets offer the herbalist a useful lymphatic remedy that can help soothe stuck and stagnant congestion in the body.

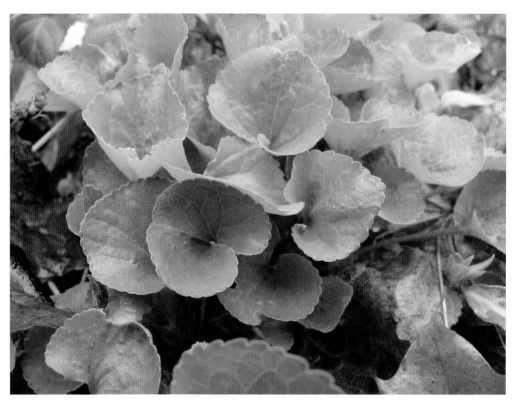

Violet leaves and flowers are not only a nourishing spring food, but are also a useful lymphatic for the herbalist. Prepare them as tincture, tea, or massage oil to help the body clear stuck and stagnant lymphatic areas.

How to Identify

Violet is a small herbaceous perennial with soft, heart-shaped, scalloped leaves arranged in a basal rosette. Flowers extend on short stems from the leaf axils, with a five-petaled, bilaterally symmetrical white to purple blossom. Depending on the species, flowers can be lightly or heavily scented.

Where, When, and How to Wildcraft

Look for violets growing abundantly in the dappled shade of fields and disturbed places, or in lawns of untreated grass. The violet plant begins to unfurl in early April and continues to grow and bloom through May. It begins to die back in summer and then reappears with another set of leaves to gather later in the fall when the rains return. Hand-pick basketfuls of leaves, choosing those that are relatively clean and soil-free. They will store one or two days in the refrigerator in a moist towel; wash them when you're ready to use them.

Harvest the flowers on a dry day, because excess rain and moisture can damage the fragile blooms. Dry them on a screen for later use, but be forewarned: what looks like a large gathering of blossoms will dry down to about one-tenth the size. They are so pretty, though, that it's worth the effort.

Medicinal Uses

Violet flowers and leaves are not only a nourishing food, but they are a useful lymphatic tonic as well. Prepare violet leaves and flowers as tincture, tea, or massage oil to help clear stuck and stagnant lymphatic areas of the body.

Violet flower and leaf preparations are particularly helpful for breast and prostate issues when used as a compress, massage oil, or liniment. The herb works well in combination with dandelion flower and other lymphatic herbs such as ceanothus, cleavers, and mullein.

Future Harvests

Violet is a common spring plant, and gathering its leaves and flowers will not impact future harvests. Clumps of violets can easily be transplanted if you want to grow violets for future gathering.

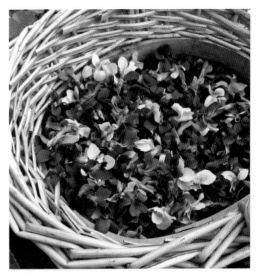

Violet leaf and flower preparations are particularly helpful for breast and prostate massage as a compress, massage oil, and liniment. Violet works well in combination with dandelion flower as well as with ceanothus, cleavers, and mullein.

HERBAL PREPARATIONS

Violet tincture
1 part fresh flowers and leaves, chopped
2 parts menstruum (50 percent alcohol,
   50 percent distilled water)
Take 10–15 drops as needed, or use topically as a liniment.

Violet-infused oil
1 part fresh flowers and leaves, chopped
2 parts oil
Use for massage.

wild bergamot

Monarda fistulosa
sweet leaf, wild bee balm
PARTS USED flowers, leaves

Wildcraft this spicy and aromatic plant for the apothecary to relieve sinus congestion, heal the skin, relieve colds and flus, or use for cooking.

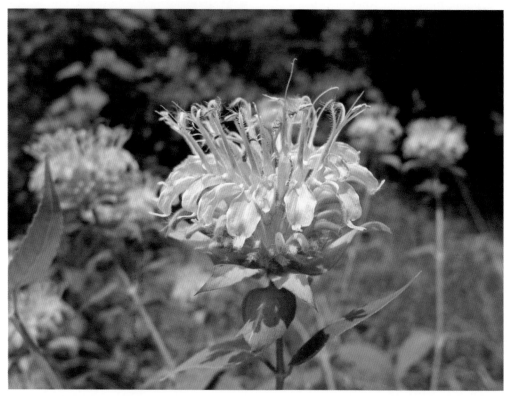

One of my favorites as a Great Lakes herbalist—*Monarda fistulosa* or wild bergamot. Wildcraft this spicy and aromatic plant for the apothecary for sinus congestion, skin healing, colds and flus, and even for the spice cabinet for cooking.

How to Identify

Wild bergamot is a perennial native plant in the mint family that typically grows 24–36 inches tall. Leaves are arranged oppositely on square stems and are slightly toothed and hairy. The blooms are showy, with individual pink blossoms radiating from a center seed head. Their spicy fragrance is similar to that of cultivated oregano.

Where, When, and How to Wildcraft

Look for patches of wild bergamot growing in sunny open fields and prairies, often interspersed with black-eyed Susans, Queen

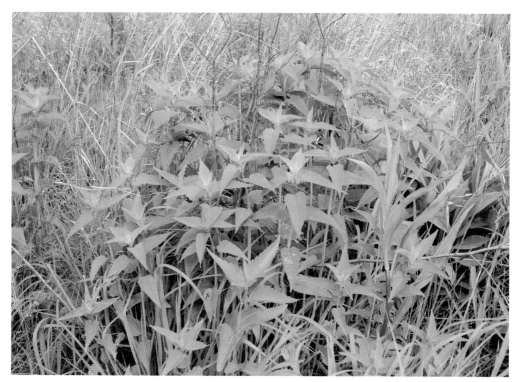

The fresh leaves and stems of wild bergamot can be wildcrafted any time and used in the kitchen fresh or dried. The summer blossoms can be wildcrafted and used until they become dry in the fall.

Anne's lace, and goldenrod. Wildcraft the summer blossoms until the fall, when they become dry. Use the leaves and flowers fresh or dry them for tea. Throughout the summer, wildcraft full stems of the plant. Bundle individual stems and hang them to dry. Store all fully dry plant materials in airtight containers to preserve the aromatics.

Medicinal Uses

Prepared as a warming tea, wild bergamot offers spicy aromatics that dispel the damp chill of a rainy day and stimulate circulation in cold hands and feet. Brew wild bergamot with wildcrafted elderflowers and a pinch of yarrow to create a classic tea preparation that helps fight off colds and flu. The tea can be very soothing for fever and chills and will help induce sweating.

Wild bergamot helps quell an upset stomach—but take only small sips if vomiting is present, because the plant is sometimes too aromatic in this case. An excellent antimicrobial, wild bergamot's fresh flowers and leaves can be infused in honey for a topical ointment for burns and fungal infections, or add them to hot tea or water to soothe a sore throat. Wild bergamot blends well with catnip, elderflower, sage, thyme, and yarrow to make a calming tea. It is potent enough to use topically as a wash on healing wounds, especially for wet or damp wound conditions, to help prevent infections caused by antibiotic-resistant bacteria.

As an aromatic plant, wild bergamot is very useful for steam inhalations to soothe stuck and congested sinuses. On the stove, a simmering pot of dry wild bergamot

Cold and Flu First Responder

While downing tablespoons of elderberry elixir when I start to get sick, I also make pots of my favorite traditional gypsy tea, a formula that goes back generations. Gypsy tea is a blend of aromatic mints: I prefer wild bergamot, the bitter yarrow, and the relaxant elderflower. I also add echinacea for its immune-boosting power, and sometimes I add garden herbs such as sage and thyme for extra aromatics.

Like Grandma always says, put on a hat! Cover your body, keep warm, go to bed, and rest. If you really are feeling crummy, consider filling a large thermos with gypsy tea to keep it hot by your bedside. This will help you to stay in bed and support your body's immune system as it works on getting well.

Gypsy tea is also a great base in which to add honey and your elderberry elixir. To make your own gypsy tea, wildcraft these herbs from the field.

Gypsy tea

1 part yarrow
1 part echinacea
2 parts elderflower
2 parts spotted bee balm or peppermint

1. Add the herbs directly to a pot or French press with 2 cups boiling water.
2. Remove the pot from heat, cover, and let the herbs steep for 5 minutes. Drink hot.

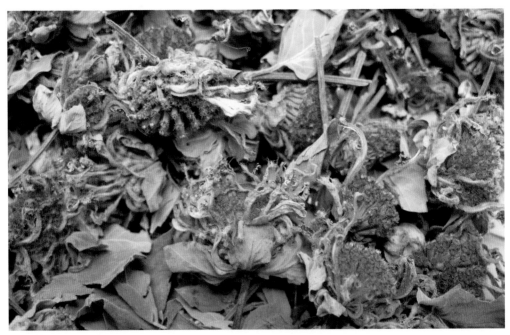

Wild bergamot dry for tea. The fresh flowers and leaves can be infused in honey for a topical ointment for burns and fungal infections and can be added to hot tea or water to soothe a sore throat.

flowers and leaves can permeate the air with sinus-clearing aromatics, especially in winter, when the air is stagnant and in need of freshening.

Future Harvests

Wildcraft only a few stems of flowers from each plant to preserve future harvests and to promote self-sowing. Propagate the plant by cuttings, or transplant clumps of plants in the fall. Preserving open space for native wildflowers will also support the long-term survival of this beautiful herb. Note the size of the stand and do not cut down full plants for their stems—save some for butterflies and honey bees.

HERBAL PREPARATIONS

Wild bergamot tea
Infusion
Drink ½ cup as needed, or use topically as a wound wash.

Wild bergamot tincture
1 part fresh flowers and leaves, chopped
2 parts menstruum (50 percent alcohol, 50 percent distilled water)
or
1 part dry flowers and leaves, chopped
4 parts menstruum (50 percent alcohol, 50 percent distilled water)
Take 25 drops as needed.

Wild bergamot–infused oil
1 part fresh flowers and leaves, chopped
2 parts oil
Use for massage.

Wild bergamot–infused honey
1 part fresh flowers and leaves, chopped
3 parts raw, unpasteurized honey
Use as needed.

wild geranium

Geranium maculatum
cranesbill, spotted geranium
PARTS USED leaves, roots

Wild geranium is a woodland herb whose roots can be gathered for the herbal apothecary as a helpful remedy for an upset stomach. Wild geranium leaves and flowers can be used in an astringent beverage and topical wash.

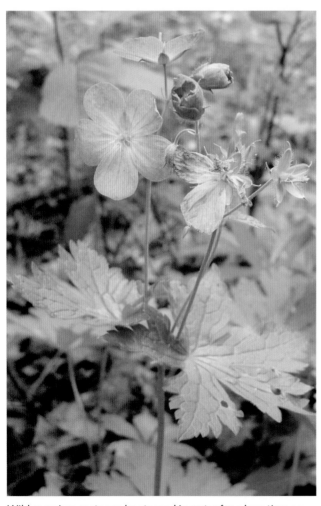

Wild geranium roots can be steeped in water for a long time as a tea, but they are more agreeable boiled and steeped in milk, strained, and then sweetened with honey (or a touch of maple syrup) and cinnamon.

How to Identify

Wild geranium is a clump-forming herbaceous perennial that grows in mixed hardwood forests; it can be 24 inches tall and 18 inches wide when in bloom. The 3- to 5-inch, hair-covered leaves are arranged oppositely along the stems. They are deeply cut and palmate, usually with five lobes.

Wild geranium flowers in late spring and produces saucer-shaped flowers with five pink to lilac petals. The plant is also known as cranesbill because of its unique beak-shaped seed casing.

The edible and medicinal creeping roots of wild geranium are woody, knotty, and about 1 inch thick, with creamy white centers. The roots are strongly astringent, and the tannins will make your mouth feel dry if you taste them.

Where, When, and How to Wildcraft

Look for wild geranium in woodland areas, thickets, and along roadsides, where it grows in full sun to part shade. Wildcraft the roots in spring before the plant goes to flower in late May, and then again in late fall. Clean and chop the roots in the kitchen, and then dry the pieces thoroughly in a dehydrator. The leaves can also be gathered in spring and dried for tea.

Medicinal Uses

You can create a decoction of the roots in hot water to be consumed as tea, but they taste better when boiled and steeped in milk, strained, and then sweetened with honey (or a touch of maple syrup) and cinnamon. In place of the roots, leaves can be used to prepare this beverage, but it will be slightly less astringent. This tea is a good beverage to sip to soothe a sour or upset stomach.

When prepared as a tea, wild geranium leaves can also be used as an astringent mouthwash or as a topical field medicine to wash wet, weepy rashes (such as from poison ivy) and wounds, common foragers' ailments when the wild geranium is in bloom.

Future Harvests

To harvest wild geranium most sustainably, select a few roots and aerial parts of the plant. Leave the rootstock intact to enable the plant to continue to spread.

HERBAL PREPARATIONS

Wild geranium tea
Decoction
Drink ¼ cup as needed, or use topically as a skin wash.

---

wild ginger

Asarum canadense
PARTS USED rhizomes

The acrid and drying aromatics of wild ginger rhizomes create a warming plant medicine in teas and tinctures, as well as in topical massage oil blends for muscle rubs.

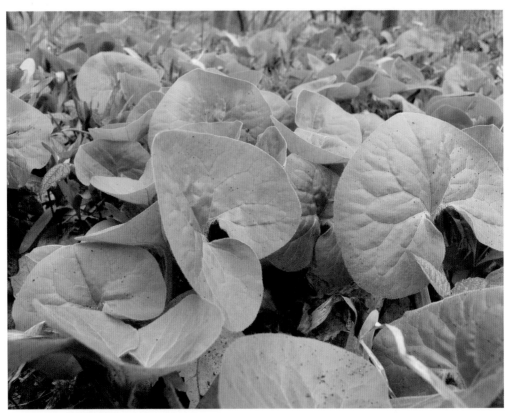

Wild ginger is a native herb with a scent and flavor reminiscent of culinary ginger but with a more acrid flavor. Its rhizomes are aromatic and warming and can be useful in the home apothecary.

How to Identify

Wild ginger is a low-growing perennial woodland wildflower. In early spring, two large, heart-shaped, dark green basal leaves emerge. In late spring, cup-shaped purple-brown flowers bloom close to the ground and are usually hidden under the leaves.

The medicinal part of the plant, the rhizome, is small, creamy white, relatively spindly, and aromatic, with a spicy ginger aroma. Several plants can be connected to a single rhizome.

Where, When, and How to Wildcraft

Wild ginger grows abundantly in the shady woods in rich, well-drained soil, where it often carpets the ground. Its rhizomes are notably more spindly than those of cultivated ginger. Wildcraft the rhizomes in spring and fall. Clean and chop them before drying them in a dehydrator. Store in an airtight container to preserve the aromatics.

Medicinal Uses

The wild ginger woodland plant is not a relative of culinary ginger, *Zingiber officinale*, and it is not traditionally used as a kitchen spice. The wild plant rhizome has unique acrid and spicy aromatics that are useful as plant medicines, however, with a scent and flavor reminiscent of culinary ginger. Aromatic and warming, wild ginger rhizomes are useful in supporting healthy circulation, by driving blood to the extremities, which is helpful for cold winter days or at the onset of a cold or flu with fever.

Use wild ginger to flavor a warming foraged chai blend of burdock, sarsaparilla, and sassafras. Add it to decoctions of reishi and other medicinal mushrooms to lend a warming and aromatic flavor to the tea. Use wild ginger in blends of elderberry syrup where culinary ginger might be used. It can also be helpful in drying damp respiratory infections.

Use tinctures of wild ginger in bitters blends to support digestion as a carminative. Combine wild ginger with cold, drying herbs such as aspen bark to add a dynamic warming note. It also works well with lemon balm and tulip poplar bark along with other metabolic tonics such as burdock and yellow dock.

Wild ginger is a circulatory stimulant that can be used in a muscle rub. In an oil infusion, combine it with cayenne, goldenrod, spicebush, and turmeric to stimulate circulation and ease muscle aches and pains.

Future Harvests

Wildcraft wild ginger rhizomes between the bud shoots to allow the plants to regenerate for future harvests. Leave pieces of rhizomes in place to enable the plant to remain established. Wildcrafting the rhizomes en masse will stress the plant population, so gather with care and never dig up the entire plant.

HERBAL PREPARATIONS

Wild ginger tea
Infusion
Drink ¼ cup as needed.

Wild ginger tincture
1 part fresh rhizomes, chopped
2 parts menstruum (50 percent alcohol,
   50 percent distilled water)
Take 5–8 drops.

Wild ginger–infused oil
1 part fresh rhizomes, chopped
2 parts oil
Use for massage.

Prunus persica
PARTS USED flowers, leaves, young twigs

The flowers, leaves, and young twigs of wild peach can be prepared to make a delicious, cooling beverage or a topical wash for skin affected by burns, poison ivy, or insect bites.

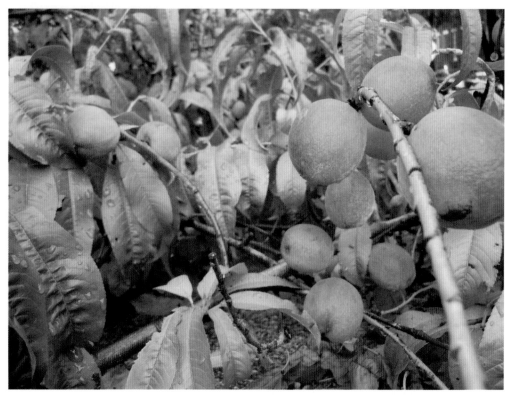

Prepared as a cold infusion, wild peach twigs, leaves, and flowers can be enjoyed on hot summer days to calm heat aggravation or irritation. Pair the beverage with lemon balm or rose petals and sweeten with honey to lift the spirits and to calm and cool the body.

How to Identify

Wild peach trees can reach 25 feet at maturity. A young wild peach has smooth gray bark with lenticels; the bark on older trees is cracked and rough. The finely serrated, lance-shaped leaves grow alternately along the branches. In early spring, the tree is covered with pink five-petaled flowers, and its small fruit ripens by early July.

Where, When, and How to Wildcraft

Look for wild peach trees along the sunny edges of woodlands and along trails. Many wild peach trees are remnant trees from old orchards. Gather the flowers, leaves, and young twigs in midspring and process them fresh or dry them for later use. The fruit ripens and can be gathered in late fall.

Medicinal Uses

The flowers, leaves, and young twigs of the wild peach are cooling and soothing in nature. Enjoy them prepared in a cold infusion on hot summer days to calm heat aggravation or irritation. Mix them with lemon balm or rose petals and sweeten with honey to lift the spirits and calm and cool the body. Use wild peach petals and leaves as a topical wash to cool burns, soothe wet and weepy rashes such as poison ivy, and dry up weepy wounds that are filled with puss.

To create an exceptional skin relief spray, extract peach leaves and petals in vinegar. Use the spray to soothe sunburn and culinary burns; it works wonders and should be on hand in every kitchen and sun care kit. The spray also calms the skin and relieves the itch from poison ivy and insect bites.

Future Harvests

Wild peach trees often grow at abandoned homesteads, where they are neglected. Gathering blossoms and leaves, as well as the stone fruits for pies, will not affect future harvests.

Cautions, Concerns, and Considerations

The leaves and pits of the peach contain high amounts of hydrocyanic acid. Based on the traditional use of the plant, reasonable consumption of the flowers, leaves, and young twigs for medicine-making should not harm humans.

HERBAL PREPARATIONS

Wild peach leaf tea
Cold infusion
Drink ½ cup as needed.

Wild peach leaf and flower tincture
1 part fresh leaves and petals, chopped
2 parts menstruum (50 percent alcohol, 50 percent distilled water)
Take 15–20 drops.

Wild peach leaf and flower–infused vinegar
1 part fresh leaves and petals, chopped
2 parts raw apple cider vinegar
Use topically as a skin wash or as a base for salad dressing.

wild yam

Dioscorea villosa
PARTS USED rhizomes

Wild yam is an antispasmodic that calms muscle cramping of the digestive and reproductive systems.

How to Identify
Wild yam is a thin vine, 5–30 feet long, that twists and climbs over plants and trees along the edges of woodland areas. Heart-shaped,

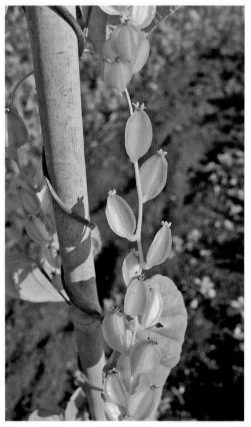

Wild yam is an antispasmodic that can calm smooth muscle cramping of the digestive and reproductive system. It works well with the convulsing cramps from nausea or with menstrual cramping.

hairy leaves have prominent veins down the center and are arranged alternately on smooth, green vines. Inconspicuous green flowers bloom in summer and ripen to three-winged green seedpods in late fall, eventually turning coppery in color. Rhizomes are whitish brown, thin, and woody, and are very tough to cut when dry.

Where, When, and How to Wildcraft
At the edge of the woods, seek out wild yam in spring or fall to wildcraft the rhizomes for plant medicine. The main horizontal rhizome is the thickness of a pencil, with smaller rootlets. Rhizomes are strong and tough to remove from the soil, so you'll need to use a digging fork to help extract them.

Process the wild yam rhizomes fresh or cut them into small pieces and dry them for later use. Once dried, wild yam rhizomes are hard and nearly unbreakable. They will break a coffee grinder or high-powered blender, so before you use them, soften the rhizomes in high-proof alcohol in a mason jar for a week. Then dump the entire contents of the jar into the blender to break up the softened roots before macerating them further.

Medicinal Uses
Wild yam is an antispasmodic that works well for soothing convulsing cramps with nausea or menstrual periods. It is a neutral herb that blends well with other herbs such as crampbark and lobelia.

Wild yam works well with fevers, with compensatory tension and cramping in the body. It can concurrently relax the digestive tract during a stomach virus and also support the body's process in maintaining a productive fever.

Future Harvests

Gather the rhizomes in moderation, because the wild yam is becoming increasingly scarce throughout the Midwest.

Cautions, Concerns, and Considerations

There are frequent claims that wild yam contains progesterone, the hormone that helps prepare the body for conception and pregnancy and regulates the monthly menstrual cycle. Research has shown, however, that wild yam is not a bioavailable progesterone source, and it should not be used as a natural birth control option.

HERBAL PREPARATIONS

Wild yam tea
Decoction
Drink ¼ cup as needed.

Wild yam tincture
1 part fresh rhizomes, chopped
2 parts menstruum (95 percent alcohol,
   5 percent distilled water)
Take 10–15 drops as needed.

wintergreen

Gaultheria procumbens
PARTS USED berries, leaves

*An ancient medicinal remedy, wintergreen is used to calm an upset stomach
and soothe achy muscles and inflamed joints. Popularly recognized as the flavor
of teaberry gum, this common woodland plant is wildcrafted for its leaves and
berries to use in herbal remedies.*

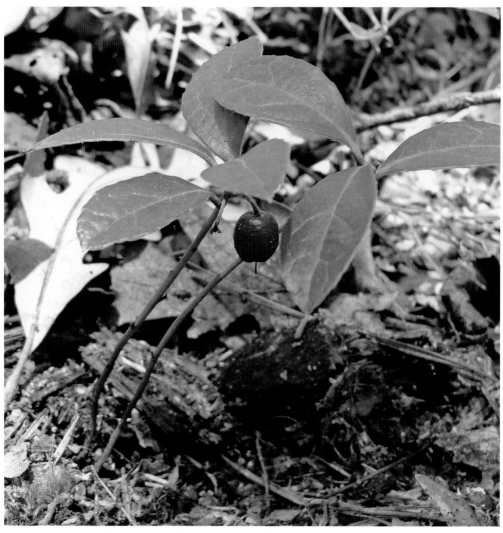

Aromatic wintergreen leaves can settle an upset stomach as a tea or as a simple syrup added to club
soda can calm a tummy ache.

How to Identify

Wintergreen is a small herbaceous perennial. Its leaves are ovate and oblong, dark and shiny green, and they turn reddish in color during the winter. In early spring, small, bell-shaped white flowers dangle below the leaves.

Wintergreen flowers give way to delicious small red berries in late May and early June. The leaves of wintergreen are aromatic when crushed and the berries have a bright, fruity smell.

Where, When, and How to Wildcraft

You'll find wintergreen growing in maple hardwood forests in sandy, well-drained soil. It spreads by runners and usually covers a small area of the forest floor.

Wildcraft the leaves throughout the year, though they seem to be more aromatic in the spring. Use the leaves fresh or dry them on a screen or dehydrator for later use. Harvest berries from the end of May to early June. Pick them by hand and use them fresh or dried. (I never get home with many in my basket, because I eat them along the way.)

Medicinal Uses

Using the aromatic leaves in tea or simple syrup mixed with club soda can calm and settle an upset stomach or tummy ache. Add ginger to wintergreen simple syrup to make hard candies and mints as a remedy for an upset stomach. Wintergreen is also delicious in bitters blends for digestion, and it mixes well with blackberry and tulip poplar in coffee and dark rum.

Wintergreen leaves infused in coconut oil creates a relaxing and fragrant topical muscle balm that can help reduce inflammation. Wintergreen also pairs well with crampbark and meadowsweet.

Future Harvests

Because the plants are small, wildcraft only one leaf from each plant to enable it to continue to photosynthesize. Harvest the leaves with consideration to the plant so it can be enjoyed in the future.

Cautions, Concerns, and Considerations

The tea or infused oil and essential oils of wintergreen contain trace amounts of methyl salicylate, which can be poisonous if consumed in large amounts. These homemade extracts are not concentrated as much as commercial wintergreen essential oil, which in large quantities can be poisonous. In addition, people with aspirin sensitivity may be sensitive to wintergreen.

HERBAL PREPARATIONS

Wintergreen tea
Infusion
Drink ¼ cup as needed.

Wintergreen tincture
1 part fresh leaves and berries
2 parts menstruum (50 percent alcohol,
    50 percent distilled water)
Take 5–10 drops as needed.

Wintergreen-infused oil
1 part fresh leaves and berries
2 parts oil
Use for massage.

witch hazel

Hamamelis virginiana
PARTS USED flowers, leaves, twigs

Witch hazel is an astringent plant that is helpful for tightening and toning the skin.

How to Identify

Witch hazel is a native deciduous shrub that can grow to 30 feet tall, with a similar spread. Its branching trunk has smooth, gray bark. Green, oblong to obovate leaves have wavy margins.

Witch hazel is the last flower to bloom in the woods, usually from October to December, with clusters of small, fragrant yellow flowers, each with four crinkly, ribbon-shaped petals. Fruits are greenish seed capsules that become woody with age, maturing to light brown.

Where, When, and How to Wildcraft

In the late fall, head into woodland areas, along forest margins and stream banks, to seek out witch hazel in bloom to wildcraft for the apothecary. Gather the flowers, leaves, and twig tips. Use witch hazel fresh, or dry the plant material for later use.

Medicinal Uses

When applied to the skin, astringent witch hazel tea or a vinegar infusion tightens and tones tissues. It can also be used as an astringent wound wash. Add either infusion

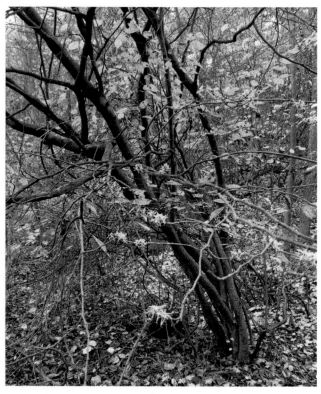

Witch hazel is the last flower to bloom in the woods, with its small yellow flowers blooming from late fall into early winter.

to a cool, damp cloth to apply as a poultice to soothe hemorrhoids.

Future Harvests

Wildcrafting the flowers, leaves, and new branch tips in moderation will do little to impact future harvests. Witch hazel can easily be incorporated into a permaculture plan and is an attractive addition to the garden.

Witch Hazel Tonic

When prepared as a distilled tonic, witch hazel can help tighten and tone skin tissues.

To make a tonic, add equal parts chopped witch hazel flowers, leaves, and twigs to a large pot, and then cover the plant parts with distilled water.

Cover the pot and bring the water to a boil, simmering the mixture over several hours while adding just enough water to keep the plant material covered. After 6 to 8 hours, remove the pot and cool and strain the liquid into a bottle. Store it in the refrigerator.

Apply the tonic to skin to tighten and tone facial tissues, or apply it to a cool, damp cloth to use as a poultice for hemorrhoids.

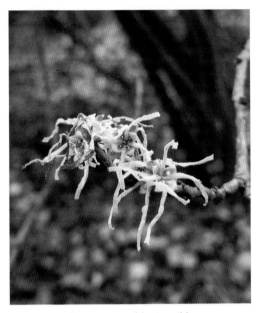

Witch hazel flowers resemble tiny ribbons.

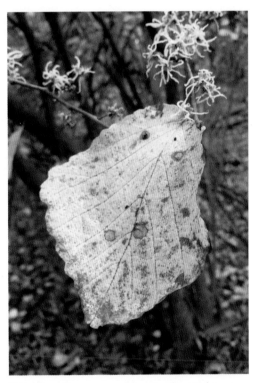

Witch hazel has green, oblong to obovate leaves with wavy margins; they turn golden yellow in fall.

HERBAL PREPARATIONS

Witch hazel tea
Infusion
Drink ¼ cup as needed, or use topically as a skin wash.

Witch hazel–infused vinegar
1 part fresh flowers, leaves, and twigs, chopped
2 parts raw apple cider vinegar
Use topically as a skin wash.

wood betony

Stachys officinalis
common hedgenettle, bishop's wort
PARTS USED flowers, leaves

Wood betony helps reduce tense thinking patterns, eases head and neck tension, and helps stimulate stagnant digestion that may come with excess stress.

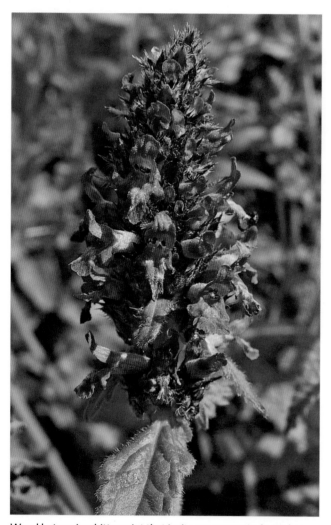

Wood betony is a bitter mint that isn't very aromatic, but it has a nice flavor when chewed or used as a tea. A relaxant herb for tension headache caused by heat and stress, it is particularly good for people who are excessively cerebral.

How to Identify

Wood betony is a perennial grassland herb that grows 12–24 inches tall. Soft, fuzzy, lance-shaped, and slightly wrinkled leaves are produced on upright stems. Two-lipped flowers bloom on a taller stalk in mid-June in clusters of purple calyxes. The entire plant lacks aroma and is predominantly bitter in flavor.

Where, When, and How to Wildcraft

Wood betony is a perennial plant that is not native to North America. Wild wood betony populations have been introduced to nonnative regions, however, where they have spread outside cultivated gardens. Look for them in disturbed places along the edges of woodlands. Wildcraft the leaves and flower stalks in midsummer and use them fresh or dry them for later use.

Medicinal Uses

Wood betony is a bitter mint that is not very aromatic, but it has a balanced bitter flavor when chewed or used in tea as a digestif or aperitif. This relaxant herb can help ease tension headaches caused by heat and stress, and it is particularly good for those who are excessively cerebral. Wood betony can work well with blue vervain, lemon balm, and tulip poplar in tincture blends for a well-rounded tension reliever.

Wood betony helps relax thinking patterns, particularly by incurring a "bitter shudder" similar to the effect of blue vervain. Wood betony's bitter minty flavors can also help stimulate stagnant digestion that can accompany excess stress. It is also known for its ability to ward off the evil eye.

Future Harvests

Gathering the leaves and occasional flowering stems of wood betony will do little to affect future harvests of the plant. It is a great plant to include in a medicinal garden.

HERBAL PREPARATIONS

Wood betony tea
Infusion
Drink ¼ cup as needed.

Wood betony tincture
1 part fresh flowers and leaves, chopped
2 parts menstruum (50 percent alcohol, 50 percent distilled water)
Take 15–20 drops as needed.

yarrow

Achillea millefolium

PARTS USED flowers, leaves

Yarrow is a powerful plant that can help stop bleeding of wounds and help dispel stagnant blood in bruises. It is also used as a bitter tonic that stimulates the peripheral immune system during colds and flus.

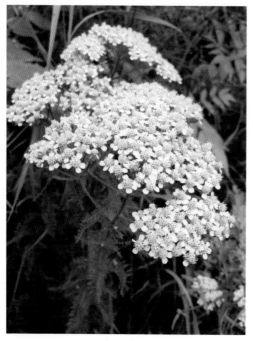

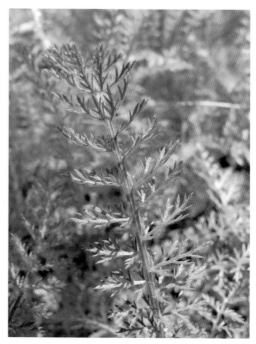

Yarrow can help stop bleeding and can help dispel stagnant blood in bruises. Used as a bitter tonic, it can help stimulate the peripheral immune system during colds and flus.

Yarrow's leaves appear fine and hairy, but the lance-shaped leaves are cut into many small segments. The finely divided leaves are an aid to identification, and are how yarrow got its species name, *millefolium*, or thousand leaves.

How to Identify

Yarrow is an herbaceous perennial that grows 2–3 feet tall on erect stems. The lance-shaped, hair-covered leaves are divided into many small, feathery segments. They are highly aromatic with a strong and sweet scent, are silver-gray in color, and grow from a basal rosette to a spiral arrangement up the stem. The finely divided appearance of the leaves is an aid to identification, and this explains how yarrow got its species name, which means thousand leaves. Yarrow flowers and leaves are bitter in flavor.

A flat-topped inflorescence comprises many five-petaled ray-and-disk flowers in a variety of colors, from white, to pinkish white, to purple. Cultivars of yarrow that are

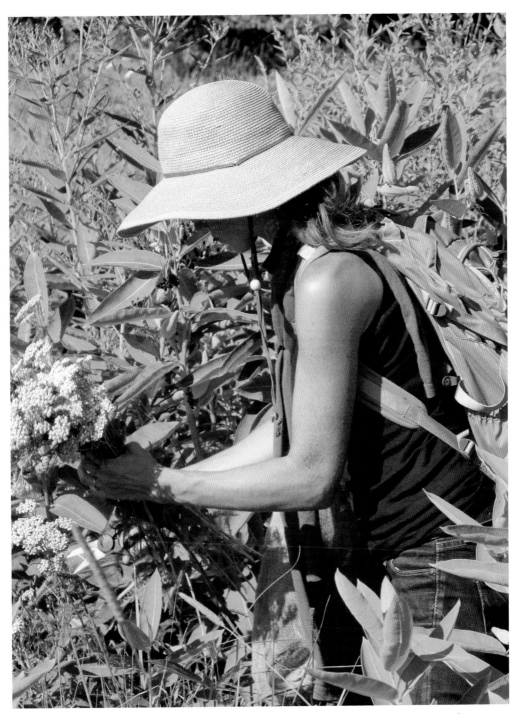

Yarrow should be wildcrafted when it is in full bloom at the height of summer. It blooms around summer solstice and continues to bloom through the end of July.

deep yellow in color are favored for use in floral arrangements and ornamental landscaping. They are more resinous and sometimes escape gardens. These plants can be used similarly to the wild white yarrow in the field.

Where, When, and How to Wildcraft

A hardy perennial and native wildflower that prefers full sun, yarrow often grows in open fields alongside echinacea, red clover, and St. John's wort.

Wildcraft yarrow when it is in full bloom at the height of summer. It blooms around summer solstice and continues to bloom through the end of July. The flavors and aromatics of the flowers can remain intact throughout the fall; as a rule, I suggest that you go by your nose to test for yarrow's strength in the off-season. The basal leaves also return in the fall and can be harvested to use for poultices and tinctures. Bundle the stalks and hang them to dry for later use.

Medicinal Uses

Yarrow is an excellent field medicine that helps stop bleeding. Prepare the fresh leaves and flowers in a poultice, or keep a bottle of yarrow tincture in your first aid kit. Apply either topically to help stanch a bleeding wound. Keep a bottle in the kitchen if you are like me and prone to small nicks and cuts while cooking.

Yarrow can also help dispel stagnant blood in bruises. An ointment made of yarrow is wonderful to use as a bruise rub (comparable to arnica). A tincture works equally well as a topical liniment. Use yarrow in combination with goldenrod, mullein, and St. John's wort to support healing of musculoskeletal injuries, particularly bruises and bursitis.

Yarrow is used in both Western herbalism and traditional Chinese medicine as a bitter

tonic (tincture or tea) because of its flavor. It helps stimulate stagnant, sluggish digestion.

It is also known to help stimulate the peripheral immune system during colds and flus, and it blends well with boneset, echinacea, elderflower, spotted bee balm, and wild bergamot in a tea or in tincture, especially when used to support a fever in response to a cold or flu virus. Only a small amount of yarrow (about 1 tablespoon in 2 cups water) is needed for tea, because its bitter notes can be overpowering, rendering a strong blend nearly undrinkable.

Future Harvests

Yarrow is a perennial wildflower. Harvest only the basal leaves or a stalk or two from each plant to ensure that it will regrow each year to be enjoyed by the next wildcrafter.

HERBAL PREPARATIONS

Yarrow tea
Infusion
Drink ¼ cup.

Yarrow tincture
1 part fresh flowers and leaves, chopped
2 parts menstruum (50 percent alcohol,
   50 percent distilled water)
or
1 part dry flowers and leaves, chopped
4 parts menstruum (50 percent alcohol,
   50 percent distilled water)
Take 15 drops as needed, or use topically as a liniment.

Yarrow-infused oil
1 part fresh flowers and leaves, chopped
2 parts oil
Use for massage.

---

yellow birch

Betula alleghaniensis
PARTS USED bark, leaf buds, leaves, sap, twigs

*Yellow birch offers its bark and leaves to create aromatic teas to ward off a chill
and to make a massage oil that is soothing to sore muscles and arthritic joints.*

How to Identify

Of the various *Betula* species,
yellow birch is most abundant
across the Midwest. It is a
fast-growing deciduous hardwood that reaches 65 feet or
more at maturity, often growing near lakes and streams
and throughout the urban
landscape.

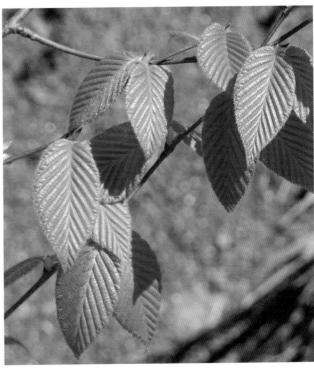

The smooth bark is a pale
yellow-bronze or gold in color
and is scored horizontally with
lenticels. Its outer layers often
peel into thin, papery strips,
which give the trunk a shaggy
appearance. The bark of older
trees is gray and can develop
ragged strips that curl or loosen
along the edges.

Leaves are ovate and
serrated, 2½ to 5 inches long,
and arranged alternately on the
branches. The flowers, which are

The tender new branches and leaves of yellow birch smell and
taste similar to wintergreen.

catkins, grow on both male and female trees
and form in late winter before the leaves break
open from their resinous buds. Male catkins
are pendulous, and female catkins are erect.

An easy way to identify the tree is by the
distinct wintergreen scent and flavor of tender
new branches and leaves. If you note an
almond flavor in the branches, you have most
likely discovered a cherry tree (*Prunus* species), which also has shiny bark with lenticels.

Yellow birch is a host for the popular chaga
mushroom.

Where, When, and How to Wildcraft

Look for yellow birch growing in rich, well-
drained soils, particularly near streams and
rivers. It is also commonly used in urban
landscaping.

Wildcraft the bark and small twigs and
branches in the early spring, when the sap

A Sweet Harvest: Making Sap into Syrup

Yellow birch and maple syrups are very useful in the home apothecary. Lower on the glycemic index than cane sugar, these syrups can be used as a base to help make herb-infused simple syrups, to preserve elixirs, and to create herbal throat lozenges.

The length of the sap season varies from year to year according to the weather—it's usually from four to six weeks—but toward the end of the season, the quality and viscosity of the sap decreases considerably.

To collect yellow birch sap, your first task is to identify trees of the appropriate size and age for tapping. Select trees that are at least 6–8 inches in diameter. Not only should the trees be of the proper size, but it's also helpful to choose trees that are close to where you will be processing the sap, because hauling it, storing it, and boiling it down are quite the operation.

After the trees are tapped, collect the sap and deliver it to an established sugar shack. (Search for local farms and nature centers across the Midwest to find one nearest you.) If you cannot find a sugar shack in your area, you can build a temporary sap boiler outside to boil down the sap into syrup. Boiling off the water from the sap is a lengthy process that releases a lot of moisture into the air, so don't do it in your kitchen!

After the sap is boiled down into syrup, pour it into sterile bottles and can it as you would jams or preserves using a water bath, or store it in the refrigerator. When properly stored, syrup can be used for a year or more.

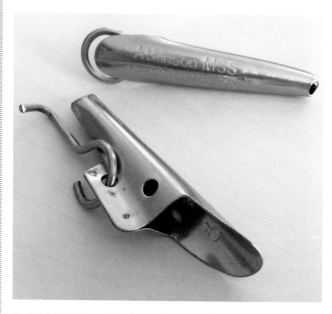

Tools of the trade: spiles for tapping trees for syrup.

is flowing and the wintergreen flavors are most prominent. Using pruning shears or clippers, snip off the tender spring growth, leaf buds, and leaves, and then dry them for tea. Store these in an airtight container to preserve the flavor; the volatile oils are prone to evaporation.

Collect the tree sap in the late winter at the same time the sap of the sugar maple begins to flow, around late January to early February in most of the Midwest. Seek out stands and select trees that are at least 6–8 inches in diameter for tapping. An abundance of yellow birch sap is needed to be boiled

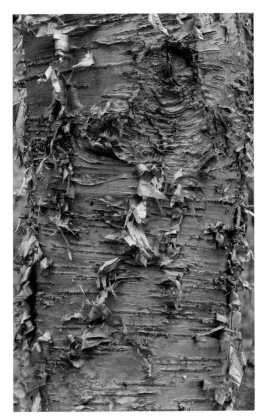

The outer layers of bark on older trees often peel into thin, curly strips.

down into usable syrup: it takes more than 60 gallons of sap from the birch to produce 1 gallon of birch syrup. (This is 20 gallons more than the amount of maple sap needed for a gallon of maple syrup.)

Medicinal Uses

Use the small twigs and branches in an aromatic and flavorful herbal tea. Combine the warming wintergreen flavor with spicy aspen bark, spicebush, and wild ginger to create a tea that wards off a chill and stimulates digestion.

Small twigs and branches can also be infused in oil to use as a soothing musculoskeletal massage oil or salve. Blend birch with resinous poplar buds or goldenrod, St. John's wort, and yarrow to soothe sore muscles and aching joints. Boil the tree sap and prepare it as syrup (in the same way maple syrup is processed) to use in the apothecary as an ingredient for elixirs.

Future Harvests

Yellow birch is a fast-growing tree that is abundant throughout the Midwest. Wildcraft bark and twigs from smaller saplings or from fallen branches. Tapping mature trees and harvesting the tips of branches in moderation are both sustainable harvesting strategies that will not harm the trees.

HERBAL PREPARATIONS

Yellow birch tea
Infusion
Drink ½ cup.

Yellow birch tincture
1 part fresh bark, leaves, and twigs, chopped
2 parts menstruum (95 percent alcohol,
  5 percent distilled water)
or
1 part dry bark, leaves, and twigs, chopped
4 parts menstruum (95 percent alcohol,
  5 percent distilled water)
Take 10–15 drops as needed.

Yellow birch–infused oil
1 part fresh bark, leaves, and twigs, chopped
2 parts oil
or
1 part dry bark, leaves, and twigs, chopped
4 parts oil
Use for massage.

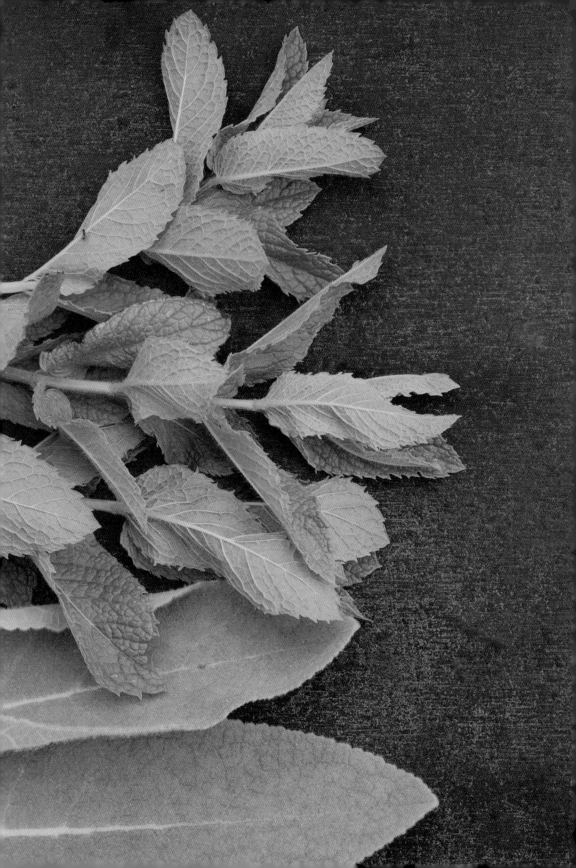

METRIC CONVERSIONS

INCHES	CENTIMETERS		FEET	METERS
¼	0.6		1	0.3
⅜	1.0		2	0.6
½	1.3		3	0.9
¾	1.9		4	1.2
1	2.5		5	1.5
2	5.1		6	1.8
3	7.6		7	2.1
4	10.0		8	2.4
5	12.7		9	2.7
6	15.2		10	3
7	17.8			
8	20.3			
9	22.9			
10	25.4			

TO CONVERT LENGTH:	MULTIPLY BY
Yards to meters	0.90
Inches to centimeters	2.54
Inches to millimeters	25.40
Feet to centimeters	30.50

TEMPERATURES

Degrees Celsius = 5/9 × (degrees Fahrenheit – 32)

Degrees Fahrenheit = (9/5 × degrees Celsius) + 32

SUGGESTED FURTHER READING

Much of my learning has come from direct, hands-on experience, and I cannot emphasize enough how much you can learn just by spending time with plants in the field and in the kitchen. In addition to gaining hands-on experience, I encourage you to grow your own plant library to include field guides, recipe books, and nature writings. Here are a few books from my herbal library that you may find useful on your own learning journey.

RECOMMENDED READING

Barron, George. *Mushrooms of Northeast North America: Midwest to New England.* Auburn, WA: Lone Pine Publishing. 1999.

Christopher, John. *School of Natural Healing.* Provo, UT: BiWorld Publishers, Inc. 1976.

Davidow, Joie. *Infusions of Healing: A Treasury of Mexican American Herbal Remedies.* New York, NY: Fireside. 1999.

Flint, Margi. *The Practicing Herbalist.* Marblehead, MA: EarthSong Press. 2011.

Foster, Steven. *101 Medicinal Herbs: History, Use, Recommended Dosages & Cautions.* Loveland, CO: Interweave Press. 1998.

Fournier-Rosset, Jany. *From Saint Hildegard's Kitchen: Foods of Health, Foods of Joy.* Liguori, MO: Liguori Publications. 1999.

Gladstar, Rosemary. *Rosemary Gladstar's Herbal Recipes for Vibrant Health: 175 Teas, Tonics, Oils, Salves, Tinctures, and Other Natural Remedies for the Entire Family.* North Adams, MA: Storey Publishing. 2008.

Green, James. *The Herbal Medicine-Maker's Handbook: A Home Manual.* Berkeley, CA: Ten Speed Press. 2000.

Grieve, Margaret. *A Modern Herbal: The Medicinal, Culinary, Cosmetic and Economic Properties, Cultivation and Folk-Lore of Herbs, Grasses, Fungi, Shrubs & Trees with Their Modern Scientific Uses.* Volumes 1 and 2. New York, NY: Dover Publications. 1971.

Griggs, Barbara. *Green Pharmacy: The History and Evolution of Western Herbal Medicine.* Rochester, VT: Healing Arts Press. 1997.

Hoffman, David. *The New Holistic Herbal.* Rockport, ME: Element, Inc. 1992.

Hutchens, Alma. *Indian Herbalogy of North America: The Definitive Guide to Native Medicinal Plants and Their Uses.* Boston, MA: Shambhala Publications, Inc. 1991.

Kress, Henriette. *Practical Herbs.* Helsinki, Finland: Yrtit ja yrttiterapia Henriette Kress. 2011.

Mase, Guido. *The Wild Medicine Solution: Healing with Aromatic, Bitter, and Tonic Plants.* Rochester, VT: Healing Arts Press. 2013.

Ody, Penelope. *Complete Guide to Medicinal Herbs.* New York, NY: Dorling Kindersley, Inc. 2000.

Stargrove, Mitchel Bebel, Jonathan Trea-
sure, and Dwight McKee. *Herb, Nutrient,
and Drug interactions: Clinical Implications
and Therapeutic Strategies*. St. Louis, MO:
Elsevier. 2008.

Strehlow, Wighard, and Gottfried Hertzga.
Hildegard of Bingen's Medicine. Santa Fe,
NM: Bear & Company, Inc. 1988.

Tierra, Michael. *The Way of Herbs*. New York,
NY: Pocket Books. 1990.

Tilford, Gregory. *Edible and Medicinal Plants
of the West*. Missoula, MT: Mountain Press
Publishing Company. 1997.

Winston, David, and Steven Maimes. *Adapto-
gens: Herbs for strength, Stamina and Stress
Relief*. Rochester, VT: Healing Arts Press.
2007

Wood, Matthew. *The Book of Herbal Wisdom:
Using plants as medicine*. Berkeley, CA:
North Atlantic Books. 1997.

———. *The Earthwise Herbal: A Complete
Guide to Old World Medicinal Plants*. Berkeley, CA: North Atlantic Books. 2008.

———. *The Earthwise Herbal: A Complete
Guide to New World Medicinal Plants*.
Berkeley, CA: North Atlantic Books. 2009.

———. *Vitalism: The History of Herbalism,
Homeopathy, and Flower Essences*. Berkeley,
CA: North Atlantic Books. 2005.

ONLINE RESOURCES

There is a growing web presence of online
herbal expertise from around the country.
Here is a sampling of my favorite wild plant
experts' online sites.

7Song: 7song.com

Brianna Rose Wiles: roseofwellness.com

Jim McDonald: herbcraft.org

Kiva Rose: bearmedicineherbals.com/about

Kristine Brown: herbalrootszine.com

Rebecca Altman: cauldronsandcrockpots.com

Renée Davis: goldrootherbs.com/about

Rosalee de la Forêt: herbalremediesadvice.org

Sean Donahue: greenmanramblings.blogspot.
com

Stephany Hoffelt: naturallysimple.org

Traci Picard: fellowworkersfarm.com

ACKNOWLEDGMENTS

This book would not have been possible without the love and support of my best friends, Holly, Lorissa, Roberta, and Robert, and my children, Jacob and Emma. You support me when my energy waxes and wanes, and you encourage me to do my best. Thank you for helping me through this process and for being courageous enough to taste my herbal potions.

Oh, and my golden retriever, Rosie, I am grateful for your warm dog kisses and willingness to join me in the woods. You are always by my side.

A big shout out goes to my production team at Timber Press—their enthusiasm for the project and helpfulness in curating a final piece has been a large factor in the success of the book. I cannot fail to mention the gratitude I have for my own writing support team including my local editor, Holly Bechiri. Her knack for a good story goes unmatched, and she keeps me on my toes with her red pen.

Thanks also go to Mike Krebill, my botanical technical reviewer. Mike's expertise helped me clarify the important botanical details of the plants I feature in this book.

To my herbal tribe—thank you for keeping me rooted and for the herbal brilliance you offer to the world. I can start a small list, but I am sure to forget someone amazing: Jim McDonald, Rebecca McTrouble, Briana Rose Wiles, Kristine Brown, Stacey Quade, Caroline Gagnon, Traci Picard, Shelley Torgrove, Daniel Pol Pech, Stephany Hoffelt, Larken Bunce, Guido Masse, Renee Davis, Susan Marynowski, Sean Donahue, Leslita Williams, Gina Brown, Chris Hagey, Tory O'Haire, Camille Leinbach, and many more. Thank you especially for believing in me and my own herbal contributions.

And, of course, thank you to the plants. You keep me on course, you inspire, and you nourish.

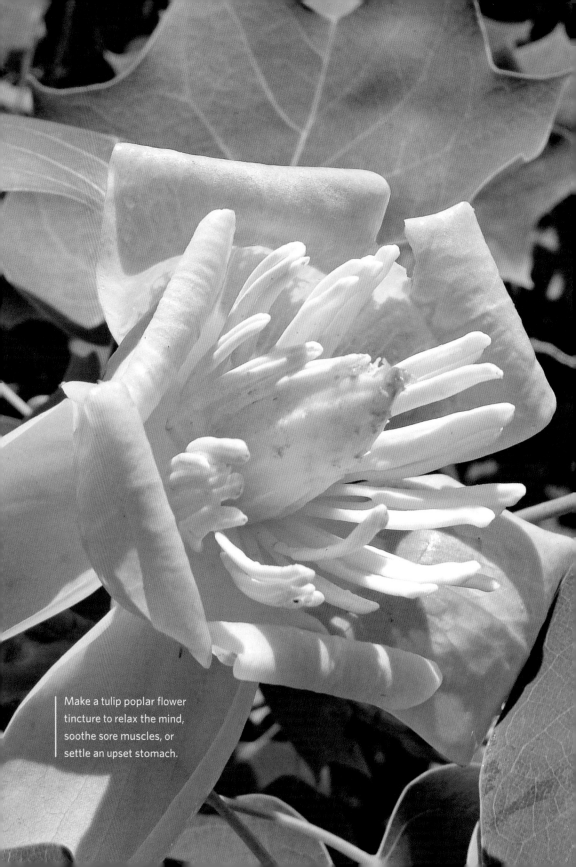

Make a tulip poplar flower
tincture to relax the mind,
soothe sore muscles, or
settle an upset stomach.

PHOTOGRAPHY CREDITS

Angelyn Whitmeyer, pages 104, 293, 295
Johnny Quirin, page 10
Leda Meredith, page 280
Mike Krebill, pages 216, 264
Sarah Milhollin, pages 3, 5, 6–7, 296
Seth Starner, pages 136, 144

Flickr

Used under a Creative Commons Attribution–ShareAlike 2.0 Generic license
Franco Folini, page 148
Joan Simon, page 36
Randi Hauysken, page 178

Used under a Creative Commons Attribution 2.0 Generic license
Peter Stevens, page 48
sashimomura, page 225

Wikimedia

Used under a Creative Commons Universal Public Domain Dedication CC0 1.0 license
Cbaile19, pages 122, 169

Used under a Creative Commons Attribution–Share Alike 1.0 Generic license
JohnOyston, page 85

Used under a Creative Commons Attribution–Share Alike 2.5 Generic license
Andreas Trepte (http://photo-natur.de),
   page 94

Used under a Creative Commons Attribution–Share Alike 3.0 Unported license
Christian Fischer, page 268
Diego Delso, page 114
Fritzflohrreynolds, page 234
Lauren Tersk, page 195
Rolf Engstrand, page 238

Used under a GNU Free Documentation License and a Creative Commons Attribution–Share Alike 3.0 Unported license
H. Zell, pages 80, 126, 282, 288

Used under a Creative Commons Attribution–Share Alike 3.0 Unported license
Fungus Guy, page 102

Used under a Creative Commons Attribution–Share Alike 4.0 International license
Greenmars, page 55
Ryan Hodnett, pages 38, 141

Released into the Public Domain
Huw Williams (Huwmanbeing), page 201

All other photos are by the author.

INDEX

M

mad-dog skullcap, 238
Mahonia aquifolium, 195
Maianthemum racemosum, 242
maitake, 33, 175–177
Malus species, 44
map of your area, creating, 14
mare's tail, 150
Marrubium species, 148
masala chai, 88
massage oils, 101, 107, 182, 248, 279, 285
mastitis, 86, 93, 115, 214–215
Maya abdominal massage, 107, 170, 182
mead, 22, 24
meadowsweet, 32, 178–179
medicine-making, 12, 19–20, 21–26
melancholy, sadness, and grief, 43, 72, 145, 165, 228, 255, 257
melanomas, 111
Melilotus species, 256
Melissa officinalis, 164
men
  fertility support, 190
  prostate health, 163, 200, 221–222, 271
menstrual cramps, 103, 263, 282
menstruums, 22
  for alcohol-based tinctures, 22–23
  for vinegar-based tinctures, 47
mental function and clarity, 132
mental tension, relieving, 37, 182, 239, 289
Mentha spicata, 245
Mentha ×piperita, 205
metabolic tonics, 39, 75, 81, 86, 106, 279
methyl salicylate, 285
Midwest regions defined, 14
migraines, 131
Mineral-Dense, Plant-Based Broths, 188
mineral-dense plant products
  broths, 151, 187–190
  how to extract minerals from plants, 21–22
  molasses syrup, 109–110

teas and other drinks, 58, 59, 133, 177, 221, 224
Mitchella repens, 199
A Mitten Gal's Herbal Root Beer, 233
mojitos, 206
molasses syrup, 109–110
Monarda fistulosa, 12, 250, 272
Monarda punctata, 249
Monotropa uniflora, 130
mood-elevating herbs, 43, 72, 145, 165, 228, 255, 257
mosquitos and mosquito-borne diseases, 70, 83, 212
mothers, new and nursing, 107, 182, 237. *See also* mastitis
motherwort, 15, 28, 29, 31, 180–182
mouth ulcers and canker sores, 208, 235, 236–237, 252
mucilaginous bark and leaves, 174, 212, 232, 240
mucus, loosening and elimination of
  during illnesses, 119
  promoting expectoration, 122, 125, 148, 153, 241
  teas or tinctures for, 79, 129, 169
mugwort, 50
mullein, 183–185
  for colds and flu, 119
  harvest guide, 28, 29, 31, 32
  leaf arrangement of, 15
municipal pollution, 18
muscle tension and soreness, 101, 136, 201, 244, 269, 295
musculoskeletal injuries
  dry conditions, 244, 259
  field first aid for, 184
  goldenrod for, 31, 136
  lymphatics for, 39, 49, 135–136
  remedies for aches and pains, 179, 254–255
  topical remedies for, 84, 157, 202, 292, 295
mustard family, 203, 236

N

National Center for Home Food Preservation, 20

nausea, as side effect, 68, 170
nausea relief, 282
neck tension. *See* head and neck tension
Nepeta cataria, 82
nerve damage and nerve pain, 131, 190, 202, 244, 255, 259
nervines, 82, 196, 261, 268
nervous system support
  soothing nervous tension, 127, 182, 196, 226
  teas or tinctures for, 124, 168, 174, 239, 263
nettle, 19, 28, 33, 156, 186–190
New England aster, 32, 191–192
New Jersey tea, 85
nicotine withdrawal, 182
nitrate contamination, 18, 224
Nocino, 65
nursing and new mothers, 107, 182, 237. *See also* mastitis

O

oak, 28, 29, 32, 33, 193–194
oak wilt, 194
Oenothera species, 124
oils, infused, 24–25, 26
Ontario, Canada, 14
opposite leaf arrangement, 15
Opuntia species, 218
Oregon grape, 28, 29, 31, 32, 195–196
osha, 41
overuse injuries, 244, 259
ox-eye daisy, 28, 29, 197–198

P

pain remedies, 130–131, 179, 203, 239, 254–255
pantry staples, 19–20
partridge berry, 29, 32, 33, 199–200
pastilles, 24, 148, 153, 233, 241
peach, wild, 280–281
pedicularis, 29, 201–202
Pedicularis canadensis, 201
pennycress, 31, 203–204
peppermint, 28, 29, 32, 33, 205–206
permissions for wildcrafting, 14, 60

tulip tree, 261
turkey tail, 31, 33, 264–265
Tussilago farfara, 94
twig tip harvesting, 28, 53

U

ulcers
  mouth ulcers and canker sores, 208, 235, 236–237, 252
  stomach ulcers, 179, 212, 235, 236
Ulmus rubra, 240
US Department of Agriculture, 20
urban pollution, 16–18
urinary tract system
  diuretics, 93, 136, 157, 161
  healing protocols for, 159–161
  infections and pain, 103, 104–105, 136, 157, 267
  kidney stones, 37, 103, 157
  support for healthy function, 107, 190, 209–210
Urtica dioica, 186
uterine prolapse, 163, 200, 221
uva-ursi, 28, 29, 31, 32, 34, 266–267

V

Vaccinium species, 104
valerian, 31, 268–269
Valeriana officinalis, 268
varnished conk (*Ganoderma lucidum*), 225
vascular system support, 143–145
Verbascum thapsus, 183
Verbena hastata, 67
vervain, blue, 67–68
Viburnum species, 102
vinegar-based tinctures and medicines, 22, 47, 228
Viola species, 270
violet, 20, 29, 32, 270–271
viral infections, 69–70, 115, 118–119, 121

vitamin C, 63, 93, 110, 207, 221, 228, 251
vitamin E oil, 26
vitamin-rich plant products, 59, 63, 110, 177, 187, 220, 221
vomiting, recovery from, 45, 83
vomiting, risk of, 70, 81, 215, 273

W

walnut, black, 64–66
warfarin (Coumadin), 255, 257
A Warming Herbal Masala Chai, 88
warming herbs and teas, 41, 88, 247–248, 262–263, 279
water contamination, 16–19
West Nile virus, 69–70, 212
wetlands harvest guide, 28, 29, 32–33, 34
white cedar, eastern, 111–113
white oak (*Quercus alba*), 193
white pine, 28, 208
white sweet clover (*Melilotus alba*), 256
whorled leaf arrangement, 15
wild apple, 33, 44–47
wild bee balm, 272
wild bergamot, 12, 29, 31, 32, 250, 272–275
wildcrafting, 11–26. *See also* safety considerations
  permissions for, 14, 60
  season-by-season harvest guide, 27–34
  sustainability of plant populations, 12–13
  time of day for harvest, 20
wild geranium, 29, 31, 33, 276–277
wild ginger, 29, 31, 33, 278–279
wild onion, 128
wild peach, 29, 31, 280–281
wild rose, 227–228
wild yam, 29, 31, 33, 282–283

wintergreen, 29, 31, 32, 33, 34, 284–285
winter harvest guide, 33–34
witch hazel, 33, 286–287
Witch Hazel Tonic, 287
women
  mastitis, 86, 93, 115, 214–215
  menstrual cramps, 103, 263, 282
  new and nursing mothers, 107, 182, 237
  uterine prolapse, 163, 200, 221
wood betony (*Pedicularis canadensis*), 201
wood betony (*Stachys officinalis*), 32, 288–289
woodlands harvest guide, 28–29, 29–30, 32, 33, 34
wormwood, 50
wound care
  astringent washes for, 58, 194, 195–196, 198, 228
  first aid for, 194, 277
  infused honey for, 24
  oils for, 91
  salves or washes for, 56, 124–125, 163
  timing of treatment, 97–98
  tinctures for, 207, 252
  topical washes for, 115, 211–212, 236, 273

Y

yam, wild, 282–283
yarrow, 31, 32, 83, 290–292
yellow birch, 28, 34, 293–295
yellow poplar, 261
yellow sweet clover (*Melilotus officinalis*), 256

Z

Zanthoxylum americanum, 216
Zingiber officinale, 279

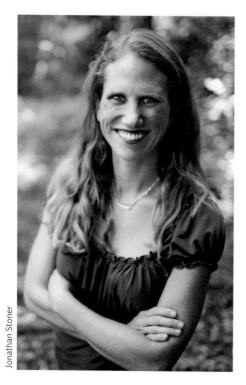

Jonathan Stoner

Lisa M. Rose is an herbalist, forager, urban farmer, and writer. With a background in anthropology and a professional focus on community health, she has gathered her food, farming, and wild plant knowledge from many people and places along a very delicious journey.

Beyond the Great Lakes, Lisa's interest in ethnobotany and plant medicine has taken her across the United States and into the Yucatan, mainland Mexico, Nicaragua, and Brazil to study plants, people, health, and their connection to place.

When she is not in her own gardens or kitchen, Lisa can be found in the fields and forests, leading foraging plant walks and teaching classes on edible and medicinal wild plants. She forages for her own family, herbal apothecary, and community herbalism practice with her favorite harvesting companion, her dog, Rosie.